"Wait, What Do You Mean?"

"Wait, What Do You Mean?"

Asperger's Tell and Show

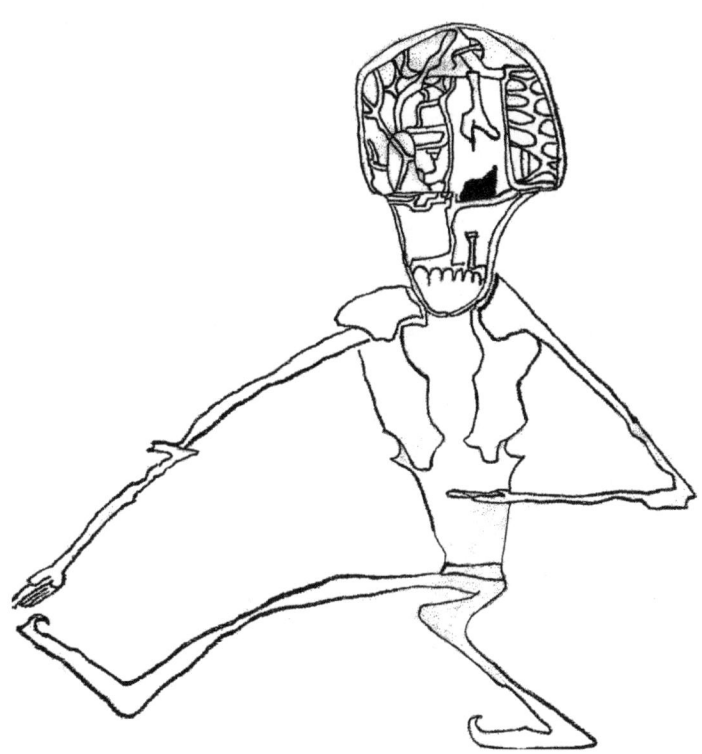

Tell by Martha Schmidtmann Dunne
and Aspie Speakers

Show by Dylan Dunne

Copyright © 2010 by Martha Schmidtmann Dunne.

Library of Congress Control Number: 2010908471
ISBN: Hardcover   978-1-4535-1778-9
               Softcover   978-1-4535-1777-2
               Ebook   978-1-4535-1779-6

All rights reserved. No part of this book may be reproduced or transmitted in any form or by any means, electronic or mechanical, including photocopying, recording, or by any information storage and retrieval system, without permission in writing from the copyright owner.

This book was printed in the United States of America.

To order additional copies of this book, contact:
Xlibris Corporation
1-888-795-4274
www.Xlibris.com
Orders@Xlibris.com
80420

CONTENTS: TELL

ACKNOWLEDGEES	7
CLAIMER	9
MISSION	11
INTRODUCTION	15
ASPIEDOM	17
PARENTAL EXPECTATIONS	22
DYLAN "Aha!"	25
DYLAN "Ahhh!"	75
WHAT IS IT?	87
WHAT DOES IT LOOK LIKE?	109
UNFOLDED ASPIES	117
CAUSES/EFFECTS/ WHAT'S GOING ON	122
CRIME	138
ASPIES SPEAK	155
LOOKING FORWARD	188
VIEW FROM ASPIEDOM	203
POSTSCRIPT	208
WRITTEN ILLUSTRATIONS/AWARDS/NOTES	213
BIBLIOGRAPHY	223

LIST OF ILLUSTRATIONS: SHOW

1. Toys are more interesting than people 28
2. Lining up ovals 31
3. Cover of *A Collection of Violent Poems* 38
4. "Important Notice" 42
5. Note to St. Nicholas, age 8 44
6. Perfect grades 48
7. Final family of five photo 48
8. Last known photograph of Jason 49
9. Student Interpretive Report 55
10. Letter to Dylan 79-80
11. Peter Hilts' Seven Stages of Asperger's Awareness 189
12. Award for outstanding scholastic achievement 214
13. "My favorite toy" 215
14. Award for exceptional scholarship in English. 216
15. "A perfect day" 217
16. Award for outstanding achievement in math 218
17. "Movie character I'd most like to meet" 219
18. Award for being a promising author 220
19. Campus conundrum and Legend 221
20. "If I could change one thing" 222

ACKNOWLEDGEES

FAMILY DUNNE

Dylan, for his Aspie essence and agreeing to this project
Mike, for editing, patience, and unending support
Justin, for maintaining his spiritual core amidst family chaos
Jason (posthumously), for all that he was
Brittney, for bravery, strength, and devotion to her dad
Pixie, for her eagle eye on punctuation and grammar

COHORTS

- **Many friends,** for listening to me download about AS, then for sharing their new insights about the persons in their lives who may be Aspies
- **Casey and Margaret Brandson,** longtime friends, for their encouragement and giving me confidence to go forward with this book
- **Laura Mailhot,** Dylan's nursery school teacher, for being the first professional to call my attention to Dylan's uniqueness and talents

Barbara (Baker) Bryant, Dylan's seventh- and eighth-grade English teacher, for resisting censorship of Dylan's work and for recognizing his gifts

Jim Sinclair, coordinator of Autism Network International, for his important e-mail about securing a *qualified* diagnostician

Cathy Thompson, executive director of the Psychiatric Association of Louisiana, for directing me to Paul Pelts, MD

Paul Pelts, MD, for being the only professional to take time to talk with me on the phone and to instruct me about securing adult mental health services in New Orleans

Dr. Jeffrey Deutsch, for helping me find Shanti Perez and for developing A SPLINT

Beverly Doyle, my work colleague, for suggesting the perfect word, "relief," for use in penning my original letter to Dylan informing him that he may be an AS person

Marco Smolich, for his computer smarts

INTERNET RESOURCES

Google Alerts, for sending research information, as it happened, to my e-mail

Alex Plank, developer of http://www.WrongPlanet.net, for providing a community forum for Aspies and an enlightenment forum for NTs

All the Aspies who agreed to let me quote them, for making a major contribution toward understanding Asperger's Syndrome

CLAIMER

"But in the gross and scope of my opinion . . ."
—Hamlet

This book is written for awareness and education. The entire content is the scope of the author's opinion, observation, thoughts, ideas, experiences, methods, and conclusions. Semi-reasonable people may disagree with all or part of this discourse.

The publisher, book distributors, and author claim no liability for anything the reader may choose to do based on what is read here. I claim all responsibility for my actions and none for yours.

The Asperger's Syndrome (AS) personal portrayals here are all real people. The Asperger's Syndrome persons in my *remembered* and *current* experience are described on an individual basis, using pseudonyms with their individual profiles.

However, the eight AS persons in my recent place of employment are described as a collective, omitting individual names and profiles. I detail all of the observed AS traits but do not ascribe any one trait to a specific person.

A word about the gender pronoun "he:" I use the word "he" for "he/she" to simplify the text and to honor the various clinical estimations that, at a ratio of about four to one, AS persons are male.

A word about lexicon: "Aspie" is well recognized on Internet Web sites and blogs as the affectionate term for those identifying with Asperger's Syndrome. The term is thought to be coined by Liane Holliday Willey, EdD, who wrote her own story about being an "Aspie" in *Pretending To Be Normal*. Indeed, because it is the commonly used nomenclature among Aspies themselves, and because I am decidedly enamored with AS persons, I feel comfortable using it here. "Aspergerian," an alternative way to articulate "Aspie," is cumbersome and formal, though it does correctly honor Hans Asperger who first described the syndrome in 1944. What is important is that the use of either proper noun, "Aspie" or "Aspergerian," is more accurate than is referring to someone using the word "with," as in "*with* Asperger's Syndrome." The difference is that Asperger's Syndrome is an integral condition of *being* rather than of *having*.

MISSION

"Stand and unfold yourself."
—Francisco (from *Hamlet*)

I wrote this book primarily for three living generations of adult Aspies who have not yet unfolded (self-identified) or had the concept brought into their awareness by an informed associate, friend, family member, or professional.

Secondly, the book is for the neurotypicals (NTs), the rest of us, whose individual lives have been impacted by *lack* of awareness of the Asperger's Syndrome concept and who therefore have not been able to recognize or be appropriately responsive to the AS persons in our families or in other social spheres.

Specifically, it is for our youngest son, Dylan, the subject of this book; Vanessa and Brittney (the mother of Dylan's child and their daughter); Aimee (Dylan's ex-wife); and Justin (Dylan's brother). It is for parents who have missed the important neurological markers of their own children, rearing them, in their lack of information, as neurotypical and subsequently losing them to isolation, imprisonment, drug or alcohol misuse, or suicide.

And posthumously, it is specifically for Michelle Hansen (Justin's classmate, suicide, age 18), Ian Lillibridge (Justin and Dylan's cousin, suicide, age 23), and Jason Dunne (Justin and Dylan's brother, suicide, age 20).

Lastly, I wrote for contemporary society, which as a whole is just now becoming informed on the subject, and can therefore only but glimpse some of the ramifications and social costs of this ignorance, particularly in the AS domains of unrealized talent, criminal behavior, social dependency, and dereliction. (*Only since the mid-1990s has Asperger's Syndrome been an accepted diagnosis, and even today it is not yet widely recognized by professionals.*)

My personal challenge is to continue to identify the Aspie adults in my life (family and workplace) who have not yet connected with the concept and to give them the information necessary to recognize themselves. My thesis is that these persons, until they become aware of their condition, will remain on their islands of personal disparateness. They may continue to see themselves as broken, defective, or otherwise impaired and suffer accordingly. So I owe it to them, in my own recognition thereof, to considerately apprise them. And to give them my voice.

On a less personal but broader scale, I aim to generate social discourse and examination of the AS condition to the extent that every person who can read or hear will catch on to the concept of Asperger's Syndrome. I hope to facilitate identification, acceptance, appreciation, and integration, particularly of the adults who grew up when there was no name or voice to express and validate their neurological differences, rendering them misfits. I hope to encourage productive social accommodation, diminish discord, and accentuate the advantages that this expanded awareness of Aspiedom will usher in.

INTRODUCTION

*"There are more things in heaven and on earth,
Horatio, than are dreamt of . . ."*

—Hamlet

There was nothing to suggest, when I began casually to scan a book about autism, that an undreamt-of reality would come slamming into my consciousness. I did not anticipate, by the reading of two particular words, that I would be confronted with the stunning realization that my husband, Mike, and I had reared our third son completely oblivious to the fact that he was a neurological exception. Until that moment, we had no clue whatever that our volatile, smart, struggling, sensitive, perceptive, logical, artistic, questioning, funny, naive, perfectly-normal-appearing, then thirty-six-year-old son, Dylan, is an Asperger's Syndrome person.

This book is one legacy of that single momentous Asperger's Syndrome epiphany and of one "Aha!" memory after another. These discoveries pushed me to begin searching through the stashed-away remembrances of enigmas and behavioral anomalies from Dylan's childhood and adult years. From wondering why, that even as a baby he rarely cried, to wondering why, as an adult, he has neither role modeled his way to a career nor engaged himself in rearing a family.

Scouring Internet resources, I came to learn that Dylan's sense of the world around him is, in fact, disparate from ours and from the majority world of neurotypicals. He is fundamentally, neurobiologically, different from us. Though his brain can see possibilities we can't, he can read only portions of the vast world of social implications, despite his obvious intelligence. Due to sensory processing irregularities, he cannot entirely comprehend any given social situation, fully understand what another person is trying to communicate, or effectively contribute his own input. He might, alternatively, completely *misunderstand* the particular scenario of a moment's engagement.

At last, with three years of focused research behind me, I have begun to understand the essence of why, so many times in the years between babyhood and now, that when I assumed we were communicating clearly, Dylan would interrupt saying, **"Wait, what do you mean?"**

ASPIEDOM

*"I might not this believe without the sensible
and true avouch of mine own eyes."*
—Horatio (from *Hamlet*)

Aspiedom is the neurological land of all Asperger's Syndrome persons. It is where they reside, from the beginning, now, and forevermore. The inhabitants of this metaphorical land exhibit lifelong features of what collectively is referred to as "a mild form" of autism, or the "invisible" autism, or as "high-functioning" autism. It is a place on the autistic spectrum where social confusion may inspire creativity, where sensory processing often is heightened or muted, sped up or slowed down. It is where some persons ache, then break with loneliness and withdraw into isolation, or lash out in frustration. And sometimes it is a place where inhabitants can totally transcend conventional knowledge and veer off into the unfathomable reaches of genius. My own eyes are witness. It is the estate of bright, often ingenious people who socially just don't "get it."

The social countenances for those in Aspiedom range from being awkward, blunt, or indecorous to being religiously or politically fanatic, embracing uncompromising dogma. Conversely, Aspies may be recognized for their talent as inventor, artist, writer, physicist, or composer who has made or will make immeasurable contributions to mankind. They personify and in every way have alloyed into cohabitation the mutually exclusive attributes of social impairment and academic or artistic smarts. They are palpably inconsistent. They are the embodiments of an Asperger's paradox.

There are those residing in Aspiedom who are also in your neighborhood or at work with you. You have read about or heard of their accomplishments or of their transgressions and infractions. You've seen them homeless and on the street. Or they may be in the next room, reading or involved in some form of self-absorption, pursuing a singular interest. An Aspie, irrevocably in Aspiedom, may be your aunt, cousin, sibling, child, or spouse. They are everywhere; one may even be you . . . .

Many AS adults have never even heard of this Aspiedom they live in. They don't know that there are other Aspies in there with them. In this ignorance they find themselves to be lonely oddballs. They simply cannot make sense of, or find comfort or rest in, the other all-encompassing land, the construct that neurotypicals call "society." You know, the *other* land, where common person-to-person interchange is the standard, where NTs share empathy, understanding, plans, and proposals with one another, but where Aspies do not "fit in."

For the most part unnoticed by NTs, Aspies nevertheless are swirling in their galaxies about us. From young adults to "dino Aspies" in their nineties, there are about seventy-five years of *unrecognized* living Aspies. Several sources, including the Centers for Disease Control and Prevention, estimate that one in every one hundred to one hundred fifty persons is on the autism spectrum. Many adults have not yet been *identified as Aspies* but nevertheless are *who they are.* They have always exhibited the behaviors and characteristics that are recognizable *with today's information* as Asperger's Syndrome persons.

These are the people we've socially spurned, ostracized, and punished. As they didn't fit in, we've exiled them from our social circles and excommunicated them from the pleasure of our company. Our *nice* descriptors of them are "odd," "weird," "eccentric," and "strange." And we've remembered past models not for who they are as persons but only for their contributions that have advanced science and the arts throughout history.

Da Vinci, Mozart, Beethoven, Newton, Einstein, Darwin. Many sources posthumously identify these and other historically praised persons as Aspies. Conversely, AS persons may be remembered for their asocial but singular, focused, and charismatic behaviors. Adolf Hitler, Ted "the Unabomber" Kaczynski, some religious cult leaders, and others who have offended the social consciousness have traits consistent with one in Aspiedom.

Personal Note to Dwellers in Aspiedom

Dear Aspie family and friends, I've studied, gluing myself first to the search engine Google, and subsequently to Google "alerts" for "Asperger's Syndrome," reading for approximately two hours a day for three years about *you*; my pursuit continues. Everything written and posted on the Internet about AS on a day-to-day basis goes into my grey matter. My challenge has been to synthesize information from the most pedestrian and personal blogs to the Web sites of international scope and authority.

Initially, my motivation was to learn more about our son, Dylan, but the study quickly became the vehicle to satisfy my own perseveration in this captivating subject. The global AS phenomenon has saturated my academic powers of absorption. From Newfoundland to Australia, Nova Scotia, Japan, Canada, and the UK, and with plenty of information to back it all up here in the USA, I've learned not only to authenticate our own son's presence in Aspiedom but to know how to recognize the Aspie stars in my relatives and in the social constellations around me.

Now, I know *you* from the others. I know your hard, jarring, juvenile, bouncing, or sloppy gait. Your body posture may be rigid or unusual in some way, like walking with your head thrust forward, looking down toward your toes. Or maintaining your hands in your pockets as you walk, holding them together behind you, or all of the above.

I definitely recognize your intelligence, your narrow, intense, obscure, or arcane interests, your lack of ease at casual talk. I've heard you blurt conversation-stopping remarks, simply stating what was on your mind, not "on topic" or related to furthering conversation. You appear alert and fearless, often childlike, though you are grown.

You rarely initiate conversation, or any personal interaction; but when you do speak, I'm amazed by your articulation, vocabulary, and ability to "download" an amazing amount of detailed information on a topic about which you know plenty. You seem aloof or reclusive and mostly emotionless or "cold."

I know your fleeting eye contact, glazed stare, wide-open eyes, or eye movement suggestive of one whose eyes float around or dart upward or sideways for no apparent purpose. You lack some expression in your face and voice or you speak quickly, at the wrong volume, or present with an unusual intonation or rhythm. If you talk with your hands at all, the movements are peculiar and mostly about the fingers.

You may seem not to understand what I'm saying; you may hear every word but don't quite catch my meaning. I've been a little afraid to talk to you for fear that I'd say something that you'd take issue with, thereby precipitating a meltdown. I've seen your frustration and rage. Your pain has presented itself in self-injury and depression, in anger, in striking out.

It was April 2007, when I first saw Dylan's silhouette standing in the doorway of Aspiedom. As my awareness of the syndrome increased, I began to see around him and deeper and deeper into *his* wonderland. More and more of *you* came into view, first from my work place, then from my family, from history, and now, *unrecognized as such*, from television talk shows! It is *you*, there in Aspiedom, who fascinate me and intrigue me. It is *you* to whom my respect is laid out, and if *you* are suffering, it is *you* for whom my heart breaks. *You,* in your multifaceted magnificence, are *the* meaning for every word written here . . . .

PARENTAL EXPECTATIONS

"O wonderful son, that can so astonish a mother!"
—*Hamlet*

Dylan is our third and last son. The pregnancy went well, the delivery was natural. We were only in our twenties when he completed the family, joining us and his brothers, four-year-old Jason and two-year-old Justin. We were delighted.

In a recent telephone conversation with Dylan's preschool teacher of thirty-six years ago, Laura Mailhot, she reminded me that from the time parents realize they are going to have a child, they develop expectations for that child. Of course, we were *not* exceptions to that notion.

Our presumptions were that our children would grow up, as both my husband and I did, in a reasonably civil and stable family that would protect them, supporting and encouraging their development. They would do well in school, be involved in activities, establish relationships, and go to college. They would become productive adults, rearing their own families and pursuing their chosen careers.

What did *not* occur to us in our expectations was that we would be parents of an Asperger's Syndrome (AS) child, a child who simply could not process the same implicit information that is socialized into the psyche of neurotypical (NT) children. The tacit and comprehensive layered information so subtly "understood" by others would go unnoticed by our growing boy. He would miss the meaning behind the nuances of facial expression and of body language. He would not "get it" or "pick up on" social inferences to help him grasp exactly what was expected of him and what he might expect of others. The boundaries of acceptable behavior would elude his consciousness.

Intuitive role modeling would not manifest. Through peer pressure and adult models, NT children navigate their way through the labyrinth of social context. Dylan's NT peers would glean "it" as they go; for our AS child, this pervasive process would be confounded.

So what happens when all the unwritten and fragile ethos, mores, and codes of behavior slip past a developing person without notice? What comes to pass when a child has grown to adulthood but has not incorporated the map of social interaction? What results when one has not internalized *the program?*

Social impairment. One becomes a physical adult with a wavering sense of societal cause and effect; he won't be able to anticipate and calculate the impact of what he says and does. Relating to others will be painful and problematic. He will not intuitively know how to behave or respond in any given social situation. Confusion about reciprocation, the most basic social component, will prevail. He will have difficulty connecting to others emotionally. He will be out of sync with his peers and family. Without situational awareness, this person will be on a trajectory to get into behavioral and emotional trouble according to acceptable, but unspoken or unwritten, social codes. Except for "rules" that are stated and learned explicitly, his linguistic and nonverbal social input will be contorted, garbled, or wanting of significance. This person will stumble into behavioral mishaps and frustration, trying to interpret and make sense of the social milieu into which he was born.

We are so glad you are here, my astonishing *Aspie* child, though we did not expect *you* . . . .

DYLAN
"Aha!"

"Draw your breath in pain to tell this, my story."
—*Hamlet*

Though neither a revered historic model nor a notorious contemporary, the person at the heart of this story is our own grown child, self-identified as "eccentric," Dylan. He was the first person I recognized as an Aspie.

PART 1 is a series of text boxes with my "Aha!" memories of Dylan's early years. These recount specific events and actions that represent (the now named) AS traits. These behaviors are in approximate chronological order, starting with infancy.

The narrative text that follows the boxes carries my account of Dylan's development and explains the characteristics, presentations and behavioral markers that indicate residency in Aspiedom. Throughout the chapter, the Asperger's Syndrome traits are shown in bold type for easy recognition.

Of all the detailed behaviors listed, none stands alone to identify AS. It is the *aggregate* of the demeanors and actions that carries the identifying weight. Separate but exemplary behaviors are *confirming* evidence rather than *determining* evidence of Asperger's Syndrome.

This is where the retrospective "Aha!" markers begin.

PART 1: Earliest Clues to Asperger's Syndrome

> **"Aha!" No tears.** The first six months of Dylan's life were remarkable in that he was such a "good" baby that he rarely cried. That he did not cry was a pleasant manifestation of babyhood, and we could say, even at this early age, he was clearly different from his brothers. Jason cried seemingly nonstop. Justin cried at the expected times for a baby and were event oriented, i.e., on waking, hunger, thirst, need for attention, discomfort. But a baby who seemed content? Of course we noticed. Giving ourselves the credit, we thought we had finally gotten our parental act together on the third child and had learned what it took to have a happy baby.

Now, in the AS context, I see the **no tears** phenomenon as a very early sign of the Asperger's state. Confirmation comes from a booklet by the Tokyo Chapter of Autism Society Japan: "Babies who were later found to have Asperger's Syndrome did not ask for or want social attention, and were described as **undemanding in infancy**." (bold mine)[1]

> **"Aha!" Copycat.** The day before Dylan turned six months old, he pulled himself up to the standing position, thereby amazing and entertaining us with this early (physical) development. We simply figured he wanted to copy his two older, walking brothers who were always with him. We congratulated ourselves on our bright baby and watched him with delight as he found imaginative ways to hold on to or push items to get where he wanted to go, using support to remain balanced and upright.

Though the ability to stand early is not necessarily attributable to Aspie thinking or development, **mimicking** his brothers' standing postures and the **keen observation** and **creativity** involved in finding ways to get around in the same manner they did are common Aspie attributes.

> **"Aha!" Wheels!** A wrap-around deck on our home provided a regular racetrack for Dylan's older brothers to pedal their wheeled toys. He, not being able to walk without holding on to something, let alone climb onto and pedal a trike or toy tractor, was left to his own devices to cope. But not for long . . . . [*Wheels turning render directional motion. All I have to do is find myself some wheels to copy the chase.*] In thinking along those lines, Dylan soon solved his immobility problem. The chaise lounge, also on the deck, had its own set of wheels. Of his own accord he found the way to facilitate his ambulation; he pushed that chaise to participate in the wheel-driven activities around the deck. Now who would have thought of that? A clever baby, an Aspie?

Aspies have the **ability to "see" many possibilities and to assess given information with originality**. The chaise-lounge solution to his lack of mobility was a unique combination of **cognition** and **implementation**.

> **"Aha!" The dumb dollhouse.** The preschool teacher pulled me aside one day when I came to pick up four-year-old Dylan from his twice-weekly exercise in preschool socialization (so we intended). She noted that Dylan was bothered by the fact that the tin dollhouse painted to look like brick was incorrect. The flower boxes and flowers painted to show in front of the windows, as seen from the outside, could not be seen if one looked from the inside of the backless dollhouse, through the presumably transparent window, toward the outside. One sees the painted window, but the flowers in the box painted on the *outside* did not show through the window to the *inside*! Now who would notice, let alone be upset about, this abridgment of logic or physics? An Aspie?

With the faulty dollhouse, we have a demonstration of the Asperger's Syndrome characteristic of being **observant of details.** Too, it is Aspieish to have noticed **the absence of accurate physics** in the painted rendition (an image on the outside of a window *should* show through to the inside). And it illustrates the Aspie **impulse to correct "wrongs"** whether they are errors of logic, fact, grammar, or any other bungle or imprecision they can find. This errant dollhouse detail triggered Dylan's remark. As it happened, this event also demonstrates that even with other children their age to play with, Aspies are usually **more attracted to the toys** than to the social prospects. (So much for our expectations of "socialization!")

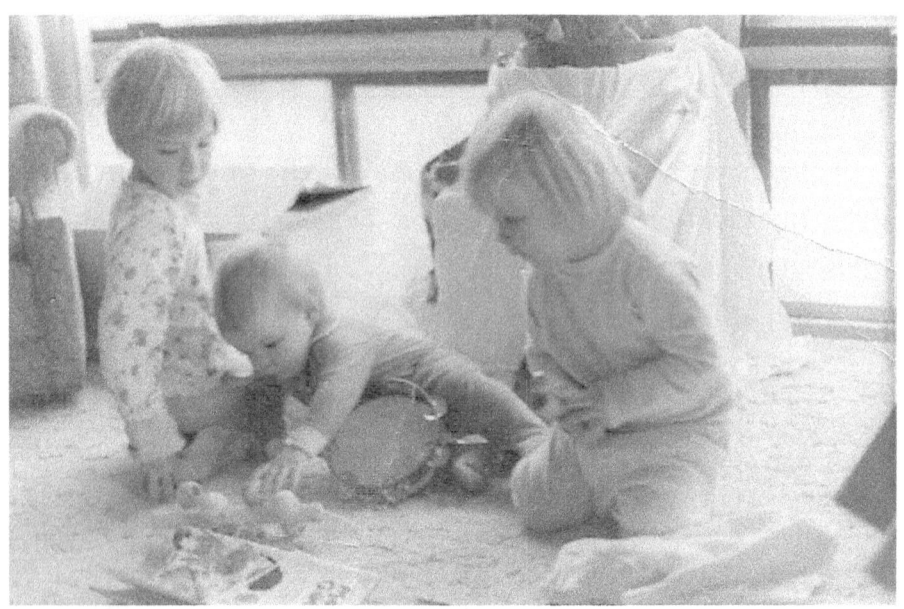

**Toys are more interesting than people, December 1971
l. to r. Jason (age 5), Dylan (10 mo.), Justin (age 2)**

> **"Aha!" 50¢ egg!** It was Easter, and Grandma had hidden colorful eggs all about the house. The difference between this and any other Easter egg hunt was that Grandma assigned pennies to each egg by using a black felt marker and writing 1¢, 5¢, or 10¢ on each egg. One special hidden egg actually had the top value of 25¢ on it. These were the amounts to be awarded after all eggs were found. The 25¢ super-prize egg was sought by the four little cousins as they scrambled eagerly about to fill up their cartons, hoping for a sizable total penny count at the end of the search. When Dylan brought in his eggs to have the cents added up, he handed over a 50¢ egg! Oops, sorry, no such egg existed . . . Until, that is, four-year-old Dylan also found the black felt marker and added a zero between the 5 and the ¢ on one of his egg finds, ingeniously making an unheard of 50¢ egg! Now who would have thought of doing that? One who could count to one hundred *before* he turned four years old? An Aspie? (See same subject in the **POSTSCRIPT** chapter.)

The egg incident was surprising and got a lot of laughs, as well as the adults' appreciation of Dylan's talent. Notice here, however, that Dylan had **no apparent consciousness of the social impact** related to tricking Grandma out of the extra cash (not that she minded), or about defeating the "real" winner who found the 25¢ egg. It was all about Dylan, only about Dylan and about what his head was doing (**self-absorption**). **No sense of propriety or concept of how someone else might feel** about his "find." Caveat: At age four, this type of social remiss would not necessarily indicate a developmental delay attributable to an AS person. As an Aspie matures, however, a **lack of ability to *express* empathy** or to **recognize how someone else may feel** is a social "miss" characteristic of one in Aspiedom.

> **"Aha!" Star fence.** Our family was visiting Virginia City, Nevada, and touring one of the historic mansions in the area. We were waiting in line to begin the tour beside an ornate but otherwise unexceptional iron fence, or so we thought. At age four or five, however, Dylan pointed out that imbedded in the crossing lines of the fence detail were star shapes. We hadn't noticed. But he had. Again, Dylan, the Aspie?

Focusing on a single component, and interest in and recognition of patterns and sequencing (the star fence) are known Aspie attributes. They **look at the details, to the exclusion of the whole.**

> **"Aha!" Art talent.** The nursery school teacher who told us about the dumb dollhouse incident also showed me a picture Dylan had drawn. She said, "You can look at it, but I'm going to keep it because someday he is going to be famous." Then she noted that when a person has a special talent, they most often demonstrate it early in life.
>
> And a quote from a Macy's letter dated December 16, 1977: "Congratulations! Your [Dylan's] entry in Macy's Thanksgiving Day Parade [art contest] was selected by the judges as a second prize winner from all the many entries."

The Christine Crowstaff Asperger's link says "people with Asperger's Syndrome are often of average or **above average intelligence**, with many displaying a **vivid imagination and great creativity with literacy and art**." (bold mine)[2]

> **"Aha!" Repeating the same question.** Dylan had an unusual preoccupation with the word "why." After visiting his aunt Pixie for a few days, we got her report back that three- or four-year-old Dylan continually asked, "Why?" I had the same experience with him at home. A scenario might go like this:
> Adult making a statement: "I've got to go grocery shopping tomorrow."
> Dylan: "Why?"
> Adult: "So that we'll have food in the house."
> Dylan: "Why?"
> Adult: "So that we can eat."
> Dylan: "Why?"
> Adult: "We need food to make us healthy and give us energy."
> Dylan: "Why?"
> Adult: "So that we'll be strong, and so you can grow well."

> Dylan: (guess) etc., etc., etc.
>
> No matter how long the sequence, the adult would have to take the initiative to call it quits.

Though his manner and questioning was humorous at the time, we now have learned that Aspies **like to line up things, or link pieces of information together**. It could be toys, blocks, clothes, or, invisibly, ideas, or stimuli and responses. Or because AS persons often have **trouble shifting focus, maybe he just got "stuck"** focusing on the word "why." At any rate, the exercise was not to ask questions to gain information as more likely would be the case with a NT child.

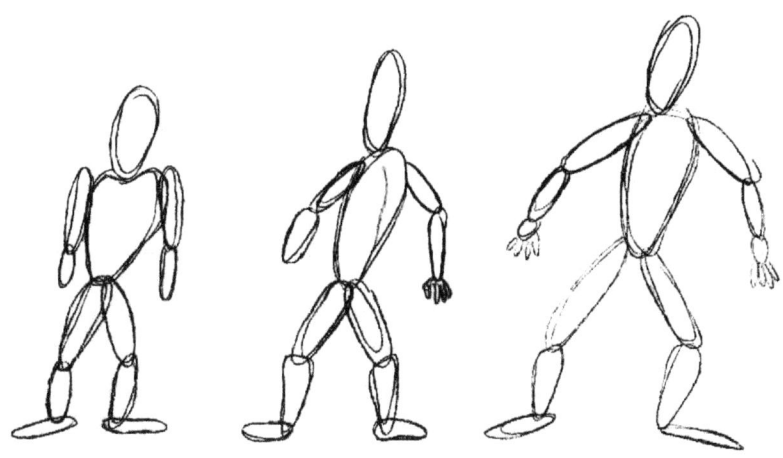

Lining up ovals

Three early faceless drawings by Dylan, who first drew people this way as opposed to drawing "stick figures" with round heads and expressed facial features.

> **"Aha!" Casino crying.** Because Dylan was the baby who rarely cried, this incident was particularly curious. We had a fun family day out, visiting a casino in the neighboring state of Nevada. Of course, our children were not of legal age to participate in the adult gaming rooms, but could be accommodated safely and entertained in an analogous space with comparable action and noise. There, all sorts of pinball and electronic games were sounding off for children. Mike and I left the three boys, who were at that time about three, five, and seven years old, in this fun place, then went off to have a good time on our own. About half an hour later, while on the main floor of the casino, we were paged to return to the children's area. When we went to find what the problem was, we were told that Dylan had been crying the whole time he was there, and they could not figure out the cause of his apparent angst or discomfort, nor could they do anything to stop it. We removed him from the premises with its cacophony of noise, and the crying abated.

Now that we know Aspies often have **hypersensitivity to noise**, this incident, where Dylan was subjected to unending and disharmonious amped sounds, makes contextual sense. Did the casino cacophony put Dylan into **sensory overload** pain?

> **"Aha!" Sleep anomalies.** Dylan was our only child to have nightmares. He would wake up yelling about monsters. We never figured out this situation, but I did take a class about dreams where it was suggested that the "monsters in nightmares are actually the dreamer himself and could, therefore, easily be confronted and scared away by the dreamer." I suggested the concept to him, and my reminders of that idea before he went to sleep seemed to have a monster-diminishing effect.
>
> Nighttime diapering became an issue when he was about six years old and still wet the bed. The pediatrician was blunt: "Take the diaper off." We did. It worked.
>
> But it was his inability to wake up in the morning that was an additional issue. We placed a classic alarm clock next to the head of his bed, hoping that the loud jangling would wake him for school. But it jangled on

> and on; we often had to go physically pat him and talk to him to have him wake up.
>
> Into adulthood:
> Yes, as an adult, Dylan missed a scheduled airplane flight because he fell asleep in the airport terminal and did not awake in time to catch his plane. On a visit home, we got up in the morning only to find Dylan asleep, with his legs dangling over the arm of the sofa, never having gone to bed. He told me that at his shared home in New Orleans he sometimes sleeps in a recliner and does not go to bed. To this day, Dylan prefers to begin work at 5:00 PM or 6:00 PM, thereby accommodating a need to sleep late.

With regard to nightmares, Martine/Super Hatters, in http://www.answers.yahoo.com/ says, "Nightmares aren't necessarily a 'trait' of autism or Asperger's as such. There has been research that says that some kids with Asperger's suffer from **nightmares** and **night frights**. However, this has been countered by research that says kids with Asperger's Syndrome suffer from heightened levels of **stress and anxiety**, hence the nightmares." (bold mine)[3] Either way, simple effect or cause and effect, nightmares happened. **Nighttime wetting** is not uncommon in pervasive developmental conditions and may involve having (or not having) a physical awareness of bladder control, or it may be related to sleep pattern irregularities. Or perhaps when the diaper was worn, it made sense to Dylan to go ahead and "use" it. Then once the diaper was removed, he opted to respond accordingly.

And about being **out of sync with the sunrise**, a study from University La Sapienza in Rome "shows children with Aspberger's [sic] have a high incidence of certain sleep disorders . . . 87 percent had **difficulty waking up in the morning**. . . ." (bold mine)[4] And this from a paper eight-year-old Dylan wrote about what made him sad: "I was sad . . . every morning when I half [sic] to get up early for school."[5] A growing body of evidence indicates "that people with autism frequently experience sleep disorders and exhibit atypical sleep architecture."[6] Researchers noted "children with the Asperger's Syndrome do not experience the normal twofold increase of cortisol upon waking up. [They] may not adjust normally to the challenge of a new environment on waking."[7]

> **"Aha!" Stumbles and painlessness.** At about eight years old, Dylan **stumbled** when our large dog pulled harder on the leash than Dylan could manage, causing him to fall onto the coarsely graveled roadway. "Triangular-shaped rocks" cut his knee in several places. As the doctor descriptively cleaned the wounds and assessed the damage, I had to put my head down to avoid passing out, but Dylan seemed to take it in stride.
>
> In grade six (eleven to twelve years old), while playing football in the park with his brothers, Dylan **fell** and sustained a cut to his knee that clearly needed medical attention. The doctor's visit was seemingly not traumatic. According to my recent query about the incident, Dylan said he thought he just banged it; but when he looked at it, he could even see "the fat" underneath the skin in the four-inch-long gash. This injury required fifteen stitches. Upon stitch removal, Dylan observed the process. Later, with a hand injury requiring sutures, he practiced what he had observed when his knee was injured and removed the stitches himself.
>
> About the same time, Dylan **stumbled** head first into the corner edge of an interior wall, sustaining a vertical cut to his forehead.
>
> Into adulthood:
> During college and after, Dylan played rugby. In this very aggressive, rough-and-tumble sport, participants must play fearlessly to do well. And one can get hurt. We attended, as spectators, one of Dylan's postcollege games and noticed that Dylan's collarbone had a bump on it that we had never noticed during the time he lived at home, through high school. I asked him what caused the bump, or ridge, and he stated "strained ligaments" from rugby playing.

> Dylan was living with us in Sacramento for a few months after college and after marriage. He had recently purchased a motorcycle, using it to get around town. One day, a driver-in-training, accompanied by her mom in the car, created the motorcyclist's ultimate "Oh no!" and turned left in front of Dylan, causing him to take the immediate evasive action of "laying down the bike (and himself)" to avoid the alternative scenario of running into the side of the turning car. The motorcycle was wasted, but Dylan rolled then got up. The mom of the trainee driver gave him a ride home. His only complaint, after I asked how *he* was, was that his shoulder felt a "little funny." The teen driver's mom paid for a doctor visit, but Dylan had no apparent injury.

Dylan's stumbles may have been validation of **dyspraxia** or physical awkwardness common to AS persons. Even though we never paid particular attention to such a subject when Dylan was growing up, we now see that some of his stumbles and resulting scars may have been the result of this Asperger's-associated condition, first identified by Hans Asperger himself.

The fact that none of Dylan's injuries seemed to be any big deal to him may be the result of **hyposensitivity to pain**. Due to **sensory processing anomalies**, an AS person may experience one or more senses, such as touch, smell, taste, noise, or pain, **as dulled or exaggerated** compared with what might be considered the "normal" range of experience.

So maybe he didn't cry when he was a hungry or uncomfortable baby because his brain simply **did not register or did not know how to express hunger or discomfort!**

With the knee injuries, we just called him a brave boy, not realizing that Dylan didn't feel the pain.

With the rugby bump on the bone, Dylan was examined by a physician at the time because there was some associated pain. He said the doctor was "dismissive," perhaps because Dylan's estimated level of pain was not great enough to indicate fracture. To this day we do not know if the injury was in fact strained ligaments or if the collarbone was broken. We can only surmise that something caused the change in the bone's character underneath the skin, resulting in the ridge; thus, our conjecture that **lack of intensity of pain** may have played a role in its development.

As for the motorcycle mishap, we applauded his quick thinking and sacrifice to "dump" himself and the bike instead of hitting the turning car, but marveled at how he managed to **keep from getting hurt (or at least knowing he was hurting)!** As of this writing, Dylan has not undergone any physical pain sensitivity tests. (See **POSTSCRIPT**, June 2008.)

PART 2 is less about specific occurrences and behaviors in Dylan's life that represent Asperger's Syndrome and more about broader personality aspects that are either core features or commonly attending features of Asperger's Syndrome.

Here again, I use "Aha" text boxes and descriptive narrative for the AS traits. However, as behavioral anomalies became behavioral issues, primarily in the familial context, I added more personal comments in describing the development of Dylan's personality.

PART 2: Other Core and Attending Features

Special interests. Aspies have, as a core characteristic, some interest or fascination on which they focus. It is often referred to as a "perseveration" because of its circumspect nature. An Aspie special interest is often unusual, unexpected or age inappropriate and may or may not be socially fitting.

> **"Aha!" Feet fetish.** At about four years old, Dylan showed a fascination with Mike's bare feet. He took it upon himself to attend to them whenever Mike was barefoot and seated on the sofa. Dylan carefully worked all the implements from a manicure set to clean, clip, dig at, and otherwise examine and attend to the condition of his dad's feet.

Dylan's focus on feet was **unusual behavior and not age appropriate**, but there was nothing untoward about it. In fact, it was endearing, odd as it seemed. Relative to his instrument intrigue we thought Dylan might grow up to be an artist or surgeon. He also "loved to use scissors intricately," (later) cut his own hair, and kept a pocketknife beside his bed.

> **"Aha!" Blood and gore.** When Dylan was in sixth grade (eleven or twelve years old), we first noticed his interest in blood and gore, affiliated with violence, at least in his art. His teacher called me in for a parent conference just before Easter. The school was going to have an open house, displaying the students' art on the walls of the classroom. As the teacher prepared to show me Dylan's carefully drawn picture, he said the art was very good, but that he could not put it on display because—and he just handed me the picture—of Easter bunnies, which would have been very acceptable if only Dylan hadn't drawn the bunnies with their heads being exploded off their necks. What was wrong with that scene? Hard to say . . . I agreed to withhold the artwork from display, with a vague feeling of, "What shall I make of this? Is there a problem? What would it be?"
>
> In seventh grade (age twelve to thirteen) Dylan came home with a masterful book of poems written in exacting poetic styles, all illustrated by him. Beautiful. Such talent. The only curiosity was, why a book of "violent" poems? "Bloody fun?"

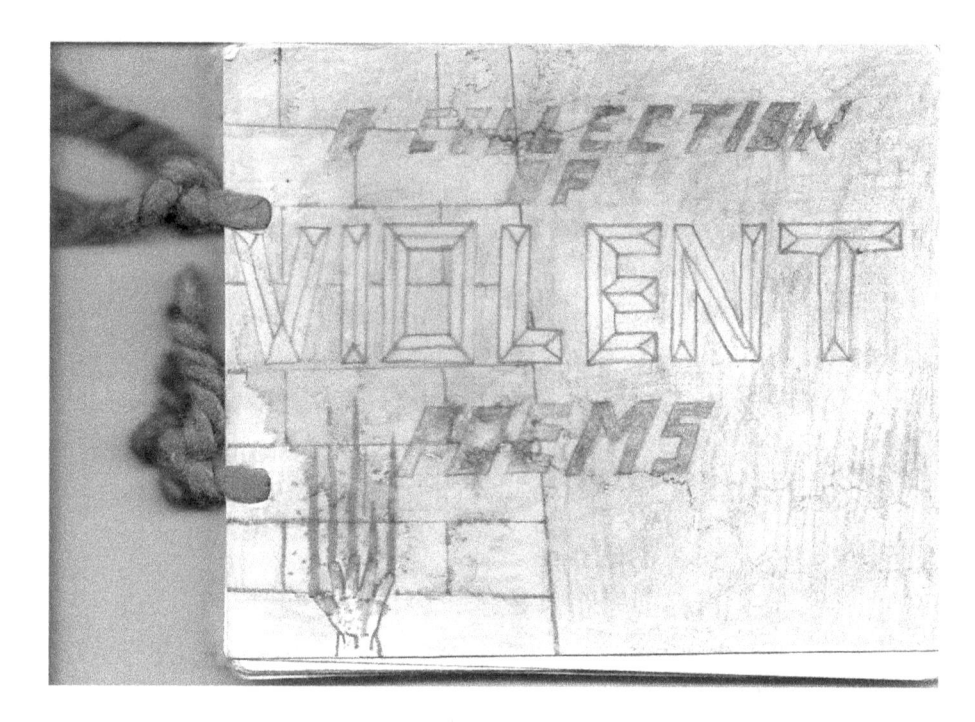

Cover of *A Collection of Violent Poems*
(as found)

Dylan's **special interest**, by the time he was in the sixth grade, is here shown as blood and gore. Also demonstrated is his secondary interest in violence. Or vice versa. Maybe the interest in violence came first, then the representation in blood and guts. And to complicate things further, we tried to make social sense of or find some model to explain why he would have this interest. You and I will read *A Collection of Violent Poems* and feel bad seeing a person being hurt by another person. Is it possible that from an Aspie point of view, however, there was no untoward emotional connection to the pictorials or the written expression? Was the depiction of his blood and gore interest solely artistic impetus?

Unlike the endearing foot fetish, the blood and gore interest shown with the Easter bunny explosions and with the violent poems book art was unseemly, bordering on perverse. One explanation in the case of the exploding bunnies is that we know Aspies **take language literally**. Dylan may have heard someone use the expression "I feel like my head is about to explode" in reference to a headache or in reference to the effect of studying very hard. Or maybe because of Dylan's love of watching cartoons on television (still, in seventh grade) he was expanding on something he had seen there (like Elmer Fudd chasing Bugs Bunny with a shotgun).

What I've asked myself since that time is why did Dylan not see or somehow "understand" that you don't (acceptably) draw bunnies with their heads being blown off.

And with the *A Collection of Violent Poems*, what were my husband and I to think? Even to this day it is very difficult for me to read. My emotional response is decidedly adverse. Retrospectively, it seems like this should have been a "red flag," but a "red flag" for *what*? We had no social model to interpret the book as any kind of a warning sign. We had never heard of Asperger's Syndrome or of any other phenomena that would explain why a seventh grader would write and draw something so "off." We had no frame of reference for making any kind of evaluation about Dylan's work other than to focus on the intelligence and talent of the author. Our only social model to interpret the subject matter was simply that children who come from a stable home and get excellent grades in school do not have the type of issues that might otherwise be suggested here. And after all, we looked at the achievement in poetry writing!

Now, knowing his Asperger's Syndrome context, I recognize that Dylan **had not absorbed that subtle idea, the *unwritten* rule**, of just "knowing" that Easter bunnies are seen only in a kindly light.

He **had not assimilated the tacit social information** that would let him know that his *A Collection of Violent Poems* would be socially offensive in any way. Dylan behaved in a straightforward way, simply documenting whatever was on his mind to draw and to write about, **without any social/emotional considerations** of those who would see or read his work. His art was an example of the AS phenomena of **lacking connection** with other persons (the readers) and **naively not realizing the boundaries** that others might expect to be incorporated in a person his age.

It is well documented that AS persons may not know **that other persons have emotions**. And even once they do learn that others have emotions, they have a difficult time "reading" those emotions in another person's face and body language. This is why Aspies *appear* **to lack empathy**, and **cannot easily learn the social norms that NTs glean by observing the reactions of others**.

Aggression. My exposition on aggression here is lengthy because of its manifestation in Dylan. Aggression is *not* an Aspie characteristic by itself, however. Rather, it is one of several coexisting personality presentations that *may* attend Asperger's Syndrome and *may* be representative of a subtype.

According to Tony Atwood, author, *The Complete Guide to Asperger's Syndrome*, "Perception and regulation of emotions really is a central element of AS . . . 2 of 3 teens with AS have a secondary mood disorder—anxiety, depression, and /or anger"[8]

> **"Aha!" Biting, shoving.** Not long after Dylan stood up, we remarked that his real motivation for doing so was to push down his brother, Justin. This action was a curiosity to us. Then, when backbiting literally became part of his relating to Justin, we were totally miffed as to the motivation of Dylan's (mis)behavior or as to how to curtail this odd and atypical expression while also protecting Justin, who suffered bite bruises on his back. We had decided, previous to bearing children, that we would not yell at or spank our children in the name of discipline; it did not make sense to hit someone to stop him from biting someone! As we did not know what to do about Dylan's biting, we consulted the child-rearing books available at that time, one of which said that some issues are between the children themselves and must be dealt with at that level. Subsequently, we encouraged Justin to "punch or bite" Dylan just once when he was being bitten, but Justin simply would *not* do so. This disparity between the two toddlers demonstrates that two siblings can be, right from the start, very different. Dylan did not seem to "get it" that his behavior was "wrong." He would only look at us; verbal reprimand did not seem to register. The pediatrician offered no explanation for our inquiry on the biting and didn't seem to think it particularly important, so we thought it was just another "stage." Though the biting eventually did stop, the shoving continued, always until Justin backed down. This was a dominant form of expression from Dylan to Justin for all the years that the boys lived at home where I was witness.

Though it was not clear that Dylan's intent in **biting** was aggressive (he did not seem angry or hostile, or in any way malicious), the *result* was antisocial, being hurtful to another person. An autistic child may take action **just to see what happens**, or to **attempt communicating** while not having a clue as to how to relate to someone else. Maybe Dylan just wanted to see what biting does, or maybe he just wanted to play with Justin or make an impact and didn't understand how to go about it acceptably. Maybe. Lisa Squadere-Watson, an autism advocate, says, "Autistic children cannot communicate the same way as other children, that often triggers what is considered misbehavior."[9]

We now *do* know that biting another child, whether it is aggressive, playful, or out of curiosity, is *not* an expected, age-appropriate developmental behavior or "stage." Furthermore, **biting** is well documented in autistic behaviors. This from http://www.revolutionhealth.com/ on biting and autism: "For those of you who do not live with autism, know that **biting** *is commonplace* . . ." (bold and italics mine)[10]

> **"Aha!" Kicking.** When Dylan was eight years old, Justin was ten, and Jason was twelve, in eighth grade, we received a note from Jason detailing an event that happened most probably in the woods surrounding our rural home. Jason's note is here for you to read:

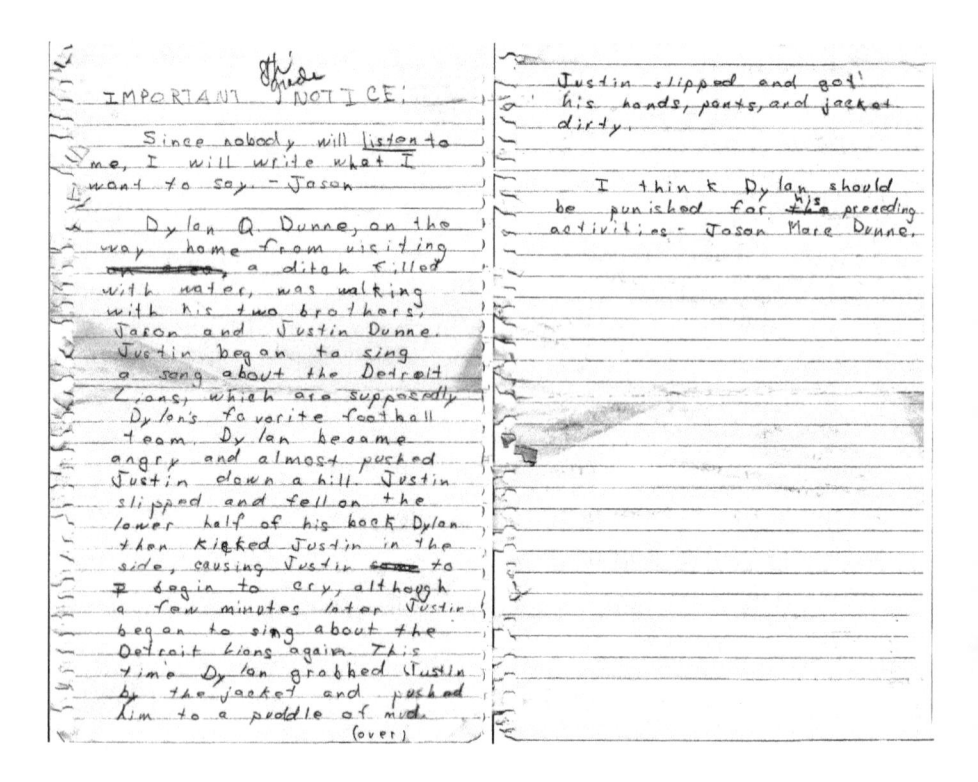

IMPORTANT ~~this~~ NOTICE:

Since nobody will listen to me, I will write what I want to say. - Jason

Dylan Q. Dunne, on the way home from visiting ~~the woods~~, a ditch filled with water, was walking with his two brothers, Jason and Justin Dunne. Justin began to sing a song about the Detroit Lions, which are supposedly Dylan's favorite football team. Dylan became angry and almost pushed Justin down a hill. Justin slipped and fell on the lower half of his back. Dylan then kicked Justin in the side, causing Justin ~~come~~ to ~~f~~ begin to cry, although a few minutes later Justin began to sing about the Detroit Lions again. This time Dylan grabbed Justin by the jacket and pushed him to a puddle of mud. (over)

Justin slipped and got his hands, pants, and jacket dirty.

I think Dylan should be punished for ~~this~~ his preceding activities. - Jason Marc Dunne.

Note written by Jason in eighth grade. Justin was in grade five, Dylan was in grade three.

(see **POSTSCRIPT**, December 2009)

"IMPORTANT NOTICE
"Since nobody will <u>listen</u> to me I will write what
I want to say. Jason

"Dylan Q. Dunne, on the way home from visiting a ditch filled with water, was walking with his two brothers, Jason and Justin Dunne. Justin began to sing a song about the Detroit Lions which are supposedly Dylan's favorite football team. Dylan became angry and almost pushed Justin down a hill. Justin slipped and fell on the lower half of his back. Dylan then kicked Justin in the side causing Justin to begin to cry, although a few minutes later Justin began to sing about the Detroit Lions again. This time Dylan grabbed Justin by the jacket and pushed him to [a] puddle of mud. Justin slipped and got his hands, pants and jacket dirty."

"I think Dylan should be punished for ~~the~~ his preceding activities. Jason Marc Dunne"

As reported on http://www.CBS llTV.com/, "People with Asperger's often have trouble reacting in social situations. As a result, they can act **inappropriately** or even **violently**." (bold mine)[11] According to NRC HANDELSBLAD, "Autists don't understand what's going on when another child cries."[12] (see **POSTSCRIPT**)

> **"Aha!" Tackling, more kicking.** In football, a socially approved form of aggression, Dylan took delight. In an autobiographical "book" in 1979 (he was born in 1971), Dylan stated: "My favorite sport is football. Because it is fun to tackle people. I like being a running back. I also like kickball because it's fun being 'up' and seeing how far I can kick. It is also fun getting someone out."[13] He also noted that "Pro Football, '79" was his favorite book. Dylan followed his brothers into playing football in the community leagues beginning as young as it was allowed, at eleven years old. (See photograph in *A Collection of Violent Poems*, published under separate cover.)

His focused interest in football was further evidenced in this newspaper clipping of this same year, a letter to Santa (along with a couple of questions for Santa about **logic**, another Aspie attribute).

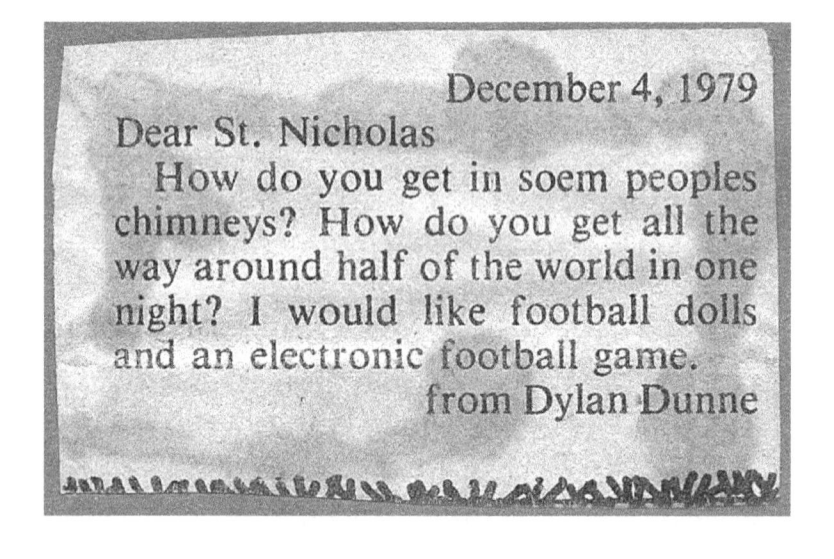

> December 4, 1979
> Dear St. Nicholas
> How do you get in soem peoples chimneys? How do you get all the way around half of the world in one night? I would like football dolls and an electronic football game.
> from Dylan Dunne

Note to St. Nicholas, age 8

Though Dylan's attraction to kickball and football was socially acceptable, we can also see the influence of **aggression in determining what was "fun."** We were thankful he got involved in activities that would acceptably channel his aggression. Most of Dylan's continuing activities and social contacts were **rough and tumble—tackling, kicking, and shoving**.

> **"Aha!" Foul language.** Now, in eighth grade, it was about time for graduation from middle school to high school, time for speeches, ceremony and all. Knowing that Dylan had a perfect grade point average, I assumed that he would be giving the graduation speech. When I called the school to inquire, I was told that someone else would be giving the speech because Dylan had some sort of encounter, "effing" out the school bus driver. I was not only surprised at the described bad behavior and language directed toward an adult, but was miffed as to why we, as parents, had not heard anything about the incident from school officials. I was thinking that regardless of the circumstance, he would be crushed by not being able to follow the legacy of both his brothers in giving the eighth grade graduation speech.
>
> Wrong. He never seemed to mind at all. He did not even mention it. I recently heard from a classmate of his at that time that Dylan did not want to give the speech.
>
> About this time we were having a building contractor add a bathroom to our house. He was at the house working when the boys got home from school, but neither parent was home at the time. The contractor later explained to me that he had to leave before finishing the work the previous day because of a confrontation with Dylan that was basically a tirade of "fuck yous" that the contractor couldn't tolerate, and so left the premises.

> **Aha!" Oppositional defiance** (A frequent coexisting AS reality, but not a core feature). The "f" word became a staple in Dylan's efforts at communication. And he didn't just say it, he yelled, and he was getting big; his language was frightening. We believed in free speech, but missed at trying to make Dylan understand that his repeated use of the "f" word would not make him any friends. He was decidedly obstinate.

In the upper grades, according to Stephen Bauer, MD, MPH, the Aspie "may get into **escalating conflicts** or **power struggles** with teachers . . . who may not be familiar with their developmental style of interacting. There will be ongoing subtle tendencies to **misinterpret information**. This can sometimes lead to more serious behavioral flare-ups. Pressure may build up in such a child with little clue until he then **reacts in a dramatically inappropriate manner**." (bold mine)[14]

The defiance and foul outbursts continued. More often than not, Dylan began to be hypercritical, questioning everything anyone said. He regularly referred to anyone who *didn't say what they meant,* or see a situation as he saw it, as an "idiot."

"Some research studies have shown that people with Asperger's Syndrome may exhibit violent behavior; yet other studies have indicated the opposite. Whether it is due to Asperger's Syndrome or is a co-existing psychiatric disorder remains to be seen."[15] Challenging behavior often stems from an **inability to communicate confusion, frustration, and anxiety**. One who has a communication challenge is more likely to express himself physically when frustrated or provoked (as perceived).

> **"Aha!" Lack of impulse control.** I recently ran into a classmate from Dylan's high school. He asked me how Dylan was, then quickly asked, "Staying out of trouble?" He then told me about an incident in about eleventh grade when he and Dylan were playing basketball and all of a sudden, without known provocation, Dylan went over to someone and beat him up. Dylan returned to the game and just "looked embarrassed that he couldn't control himself."

In response to a question stemming from a similar incident where hitting was involved, autism expert Julia Erdelyi says, "**Impulse control problems** and social misunderstandings are direct results of Asperger's." (bold mine)[16]

Silliness, childlike behavior. Because Aspies are socially naive, they do not learn all the subtle behaviors that change as peers mature.

> **"Aha!" Silliness.** Dylan seemed very attached to both his brothers but related to them in opposite ways. He aggressed against Justin but seemed more respectful of Jason. Besides video games and football, the one form of relating that the three of them played in high school, however, was a curious activity of creating an "O" with the thumb and forefinger, then holding it somewhere against the body. This could be effected at any time, unknown to the others. Then, when either of the other two boys inadvertently happened to look at the sign, he would receive a fist punch by the sign holder. This "game" generated a lot of laughing and camaraderie between three of them when someone "got" someone else. It seemed incomparably silly, but it was such a relief, given the frequent tension around the house, to hear the three of them laugh together. Even though the game involved physical punching (Dylan's forte) we, as parents, allowed it as "boys will be boys" behavior.

From a *Survival Guide for People Living with Asperger's Syndrome*: "An autistic person's sense of humor is often about things which suggest silliness, ridiculousness or which appear slightly insane."[17]

Though much of Dylan's behavior throughout high school was challenging to Mike and I as parents, we were likewise very fortunate to have no parenting problems related to Dylan's schoolwork, keeping his room tidy, or his personal grooming. He was neat, clean to the point of doing his own laundry because he didn't like the way I did it, and cut his own hair every few days. His grades were excellent. When occasionally asked if he had any homework, he would reply that he did it at school. His honesty was never in question.

48   Martha Schmidtmann Dunne

AMADOR COUNTY UNIFIED SCHOOL DISTRICT
REPORT CARD

89050

STUDENT NAME	SCHOOL	SEMESTER	GRADE	REPORT DATE	G.P.A.
DUNNE DYLAN	AMADOR	SPRING	9	06/13/86	4.0

PERIOD	SUBJECT	TEACHER	FIRST QTR. GRADE	SECOND QTR. GRADE	SEMESTER GRADE	SEMESTER CREDIT	COMMENTS	COMMENT CODING
1	E 9 SCH (CP)	WILLERT	A	A	A	5	1	1 Excellent work in this class.
2	PHYS SCI	NASIATKA	A	A	A	5	1	2 Making the effort to improve.
3	DRAMA I	TURNER	A	A	A	5		3 Detracts from learning atmosphere.
4	PE 9	ANDOSHIAN	A	A	A	5	1	4 Achieving below apparent ability.
5	KB A	MORENO	P	A	A	5	1	5 Needs to come to class prepared.
6	FR I (CP)	WILLERT	A	A	A	5	1	6 Not completing assignments.
7	ALG I (CP)	NASIATKA	A	A	A	5	1	7 Needs to improve test/quiz scores.
								8 Tardies/absences affecting work.
								9 Parent, please contact teacher.
								0 CREDIT LOSS (LATE ENROLLMENT)

GRADE CODES ▶   A - SUPERIOR WORK   C - AVERAGE   F - FAILING   NG - NO GRADE
                 B - ABOVE AVERAGE   D - BELOW AVERAGE   I - INCOMPLETE   P - PASSING

Perfect grades

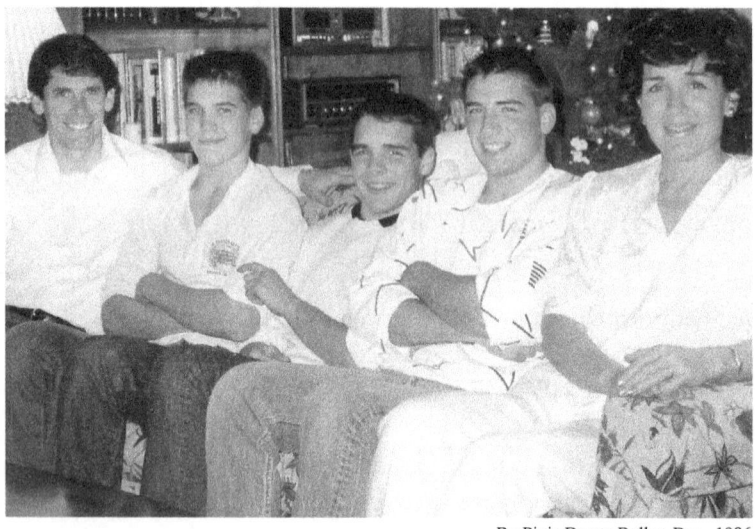

By Pixie Dunne Bolles, Dec., 1986

Final family of five photo, December 1986
l. to r. Mike, Dylan (age 15), Justin (age 17), Jason
(age 20), and Martha

PART 3 relates the passing of Justin and Dylan's brother, Jason.

PART 3: *Jason*

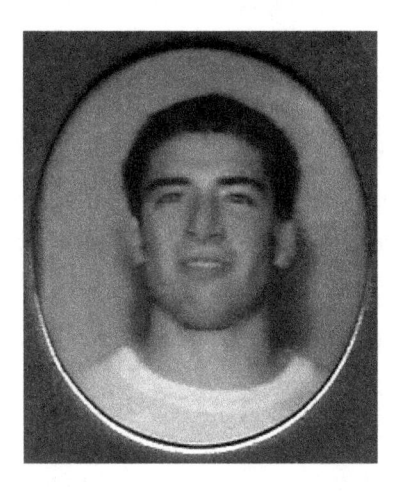

Last known photograph, self-taken by Jason.

Jason was probably the only nonidiot in Dylan's world, despite the fact that Jason, unlike Dylan, had a rigid opposition to the use of the "f" word. Dylan simply connected with Jason in a more "civilized" manner than he did with Justin or with Mike or me.

Jason's focused interest was in Marvel Comics heroes, especially Spiderman and Silver Surfer. He seemed to personally take on the "do good" aspects of his comic book heroes and appeared to hoist the banner of righteousness, as was demonstrated by his handwritten note on a previous page. However, from about the age of fifteen, Jason was becoming emotionally isolated, distant from us. The response to almost any question we asked him was, "Don't worry about it."

We walked on eggshells, so to speak, as he seemed so sensitive, perfectionistic, rigid, and, most importantly, depressed. Before graduating from high school he had two noninjury auto accidents, and we became very concerned about his "accident proneness," as well as his psychological remoteness. He had a painful intestinal condition called Irritable Bowel Syndrome, for which he was taking medication.

He also showed compulsive and paranoid behaviors. Like insisting on his own room, even if it was in the basement. Like not being able to turn off water. Like looking suspiciously all around him when coming out of the bathroom. He was rigid in his perspective and in his physical demeanor. Our concerns led us to tell his pediatrician when he was seventeen that we feared that he would commit suicide.

The pediatrician asked us the appropriate clinical questions, "How are his grades?" and "Does he have friends?" His grades were flawless and many people, both teachers and students, seemed to really respect him. (I now know that "respect" is not the same as reciprocity in friendship.) But thinking back on it, there was only one friend he connected to through the shared interest of the game "Dungeons and Dragons." Our answers seemed to clue the doctor that there was no serious problem.

I was glad for the fact that Jason had the bond with Dylan, making at least some connection to his family. When Jason left home for college, we hoped that he would do better emotionally. I assumed that once he was away from me and my own bouts with anger, PMS, depression, yelling (which I was now doing as my grip on parenting by better means had eroded away in ineffectiveness) he would find college life fulfilling and joyful.

Then came the evening of June 1, 1987. Dylan was sixteen, a sophomore in high school; Justin was eighteen, a senior ready to graduate in twelve days. Jason was twenty and just finishing up his junior year in college.

When Mike and I arrived home from our work commute, Justin or Dylan told us that a sheriff's deputy had been to the house earlier in the afternoon. Of course, we asked them what they (the police) wanted, but neither of them knew. We said not to worry about it; if it were important, they would be back in touch . . . .

That evening, an officer returned, was invited in, and told us to "sit down." Then he asked us if we had a son named Jason Marc Dunne going to college at Cal Poly Pomona. We answered affirmatively. Next, the total family-shattering bomb exploded in our midst. That afternoon, he said, twenty-year-old Jason had been struck by a train and killed.

From that moment, the family as we knew it ended. Pain, pain all around and nothing to put on it or to take by mouth to abate it, and nowhere to run from it. Our firstborn, beautiful, perfectionistic child was gone, and his siblings had no less a loss; no Jason in their world to "be there" ahead of them or for them.

The next day, Mike traveled to Jason's college to investigate. In Jason's dorm room (yes, he had his own room as a "Resident Advisor"), Mike found empty containers of nighttime cold medicine in the wastebasket. Also found were some VHS tapes Jason made just prior to his death on June 1.

About two weeks after Jason's passing we mustered the emotional strength to view one of the found VHS tapes, recorded in the early morning, May 31, 1987. Though the tape was audio/video, this one had no video, only *the black screen showing the time: "12:02 AM, May 31, 1987." The audio has an (unidentified) rock band playing in the background.*

Then, within a few seconds, this, in Jason's voice: "I love you, Roxanne. I, Jason Dunne, hereby give my possessions to Roxanne [last name]. Fuck you, world."

He had finally given up on righteousness and his "world." His depression was manifest, and he intended to handle it the only way he knew how. The remainder of thirty minutes of the tape continued to play the background music. One could hear a sound like of pills being shaken from a bottle, and again, and again.

Then, possibly the sounds of bedcovers being pulled back, and sniffing. When the music stopped at 12:32 AM, the tape continues black, with the exception of what sounds like muffled voices moving down the hallway outside Jason's closed door. The tape ends at one sixteen. There are no more sounds, only silence.

The remainder of May 31 remains a mystery. Were the date and time actually two minutes into June 1? Or perhaps having overdosed himself on sleeping pills, did Jason sleep all day of the thirty-first? Roxanne later told us that she had stopped by to give him a note (we are not sure which day) but that he did not respond to the knock on his door.

The morning of the following day, June 1, Jason's friend Adam stopped by to see if Jason wanted to go to the gym to work out. According to Adam, Jason told him that he was "still" sick and couldn't go . . .

Later that afternoon, June 1, Jason borrowed a camera from school and drove to the train tracks. The engineer who was the last to see Jason alive stated that Jason, standing alongside the tracks, looked as if he was "going down to take a picture of the (train's) undercarriage . . . ."

He was struck and killed.

Whether Jason was groggy from a pill overdose early the day before that caused him to fall beneath the train, or whether the camera was a ruse and he crouched down preliminary to jumping, we'll never know.

What we do know is that there was no film in the camera and the lens cap had not been removed.

What we do know is that Jason was a perfectionist, and if a first attempt (pills) failed, he would make sure that another did not.

At Jason's memorial, six days later, we did learn (from Roxanne) that she had broken up their relationship the day leading up to the 12:02 AM, May 31, tape: "I love you, Roxanne . . . ."

And at this point, we can't help but remember a very strange and prescient utterance from Jason when he was only six years old. I noticed he was searching around the house for something. When I asked him what he was looking for, this little, articulate, precocious boy replied, "I am looking for a place to commit suicide . . . ."

PART 4 continues to update our family's experience, chronicling Dylan's most recent twenty plus years, including our struggle to maintain as a family in the wake of Jason's death, and the interplay of Dylan's (unknown at the time) neurodiversity.

Again, I use text boxes for focused looks at behavior—descriptions of how the behaviors relate to Asperger's Syndrome—and I employ a running chronological narrative of this story.

PART 4: After Jason, Dylan's most recent twenty years

The now larger-than-either-parent, strong, fit, aggressive, sixteen-year-old Dylan became angrier and angrier. I heard a lifetime and back of the word "fuck." From a parent's point of view, he was unmanageable. He seemed irritated or mad much of the time. Perpetual anger. He stopped going to his orthodontist appointments, and the orthodontist said we had to have the braces removed, as the therapy couldn't proceed properly. Dylan removed the wires and metal tooth bands himself!

We made a family appointment with a psychiatrist to see if we could get some help holding the remaining four of our five-person family together, but Dylan wouldn't go. And he was too big for us to put him in the car. So Justin, Mike, and I went for two sessions. We never had a third visit, as the fifty-two-year-old doctor had surgery just prior to our next appointment and died on the operating table. Enough already.

We were grateful Dylan had a part-time job, following in his brothers' footsteps by working at a local hotel. He was very dependable and a hard worker. He still received, even through his anger and defiance, very good grades. His national standardized testing scores rated him, in the tenth grade, at the college level—in every subject. His grades did drop, however, from a perfect 4.0 in ninth grade to a 3.41 average in eleventh grade. (See **POSTSCRIPT**, December 2009)

"Wait, what do you mean?" 55

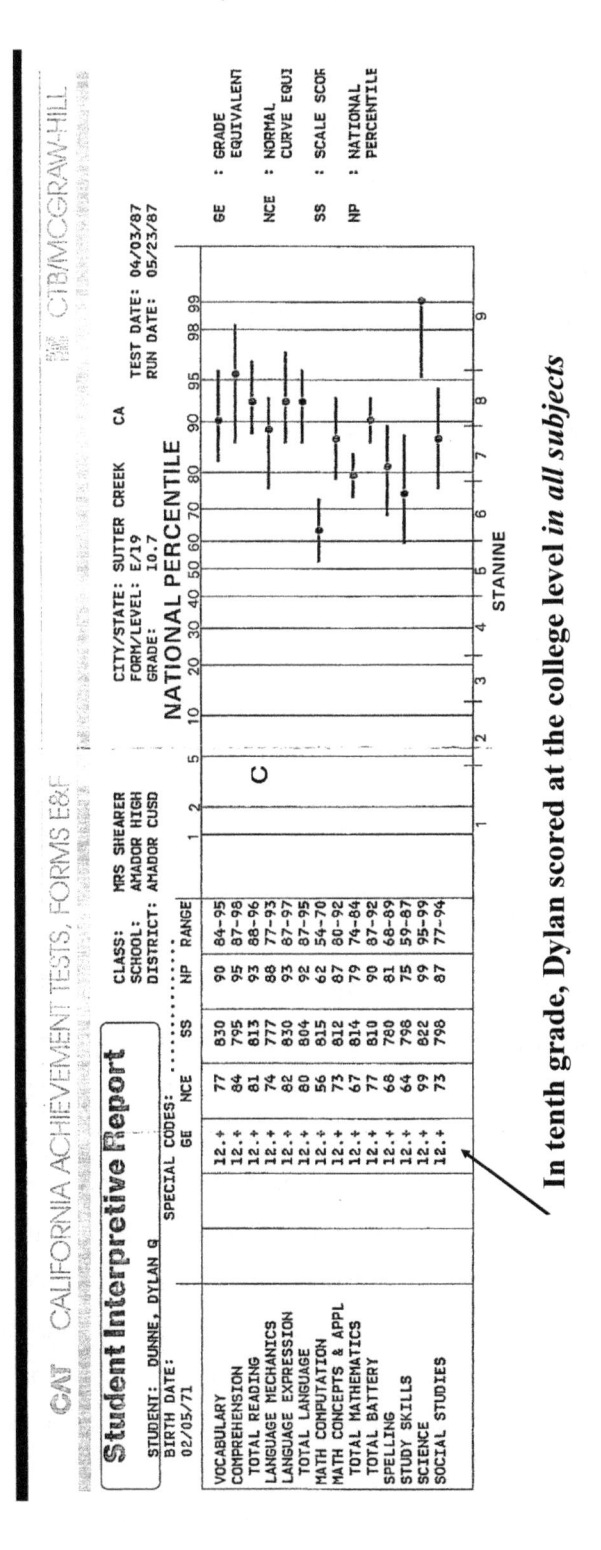

In tenth grade, Dylan scored at the college level *in all subjects*

But there were blowups and yelling at home, primarily between Dylan and myself. We both were acting out our frustration and anger, and there was no significance left to my parenthood. Justin steered clear of me, and Mike was the quiet, appropriately patient rock of stability, continuing his work supporting the family, tacitly declining to add any kind of fuel to the overt angst and disruption generated by Dylan and I.

> **"Aha!" Lack of emotional reciprocity with others.** Dylan seemed to have no appreciation that the other family members were suffering too and that we all needed to support each other. I could not control him or make him realize that we all were in pain. The climax of our fighting came raging into my face when Dylan, in anger, threw down a saucepan in front of Mike and me, yelling, "I ought to kill you two."

And things did not get better. In the interest of protecting our other son, Justin, who of course was dealing with his own grief, as well as protecting ourselves, we considered the legal status of emancipation for Dylan. The concept itself was wrenchingly difficult, as this would have represented the emotional "giving up" on our son. Reluctantly, not being able to reconcile our innate love for Dylan with his defiance and anger, we queried an attorney on the subject. He was hesitant to proceed with such a harsh step, especially given the circumstance of the recent passing of Jason and the relevant consideration of everyone's grief. He did say, however, that threatening one's life was cause for such a drastic step.

Alternatively, we told Dylan he could no longer live with us in our family home, and we tried to kick him out (he had a car and a part-time job). Amid more yelling and efforts to physically remove him, he just wouldn't go. I had come face to face with the specter that unconditional maternal love was breaking me; it was almost *too* hard to love my son. I was conflicted to the point of just giving up emotionally but could not, being irrevocably bound by maternal love.

Because we had no idea of Asperger's Syndrome, and that Dylan could be an Aspie, the above sequence is the darkest and most rueful in the saga of interaction between Dylan and myself. If Mike and I had *any* idea that there was such a thing as Asperger's Syndrome, developmental delay, neurodiversity, or *anything* related to autism, we would not have been judgmental and could have come to terms in some productive manner. We would have known that Dylan **couldn't recognize the feelings of other family members, or even control his own emotions**. Instead of criticizing him, yelling, faultfinding, and in desperation, emotionally trying to throw him away, we could have found a way to provide appropriate support. Had we known, instead of being the determined opposition trying to control our minor son, we would have been in his corner, embracing and guiding him.

Next, we just excluded Dylan from participation in the day-to-day aspects of being a family member, including conversation (I didn't talk to him) and meals (the table was not set for him). I basically tried to ignore him as we cohabited the same premises. Mike and I did offer one remedy: Dylan could provide us with a *written apology* for the threat on our lives and thereby be accepted back into the family, shattered as it was.

A couple of days later, as I was ironing, Dylan placed a small piece of paper beside me on the ironing board. On it was written one word, "Sorry."

In December, about six months after Jason's passing, we decided to try a family vacation to San Diego where it was sunnier than in Pine Grove, Amador County, thinking that a different locale, new activities and warmer weather might take our minds off the recent memories and brighten our spirits. Two rooms were secured, with Mike and I in one room, and Justin and Dylan in the other. Once we arrived, it wasn't long before Justin complained that he couldn't sleep in the room with Dylan. Without hearing the details we assumed this was because of Dylan's **aggression, anger, and threats** toward Justin. So Justin slept in the car.

Not long after the vacation, Justin went off to the University of California, Riverside, while Dylan was completing two more years of high school. Dylan participated in football and continued to receive kudos for his academic performance and enduring work ethic.

The atmosphere at home improved somewhat, but in my own grieving, I too carried anger, defiance, and depression around with me, almost looking for someone to cross me or tell me what to do, so I could light into them about how little they knew about anything. (In retrospect, I now see this behavior as a bad attempt at regaining the control I lost in failing my child. The sheer fearlessness with which I lit into others restored some sense of personal power or effectiveness, destructive though it was.) That defiance characterized my emotional persona for at least five years until some incredibly wise person had the forte to speak up to me and say, "You can either get bitter, or you can get better."

What? I had a choice? This simple but profound statement spurred my healing.

After realizing the verity of that sage statement, I *gradually* opted for the latter alternative. I slowly made the exchange of bitter for better by accepting the incredible freedom, power, and personal effectiveness found in recognizing that, in determining my own well being, I did indeed have choice.

Meanwhile, however, not yet having grasped the nature of choice, my emotions ruled; I was no help to Dylan, whose **anger** was still daunting and unpredictable. We began to watch what we said to Dylan, were careful about our approach to any subject, and generally tread softly knowing the consequences of his outbursts. Our restricted and cautious behavior, "eggshell walking," was very similar to the way we responded to Jason's **sensitivity** and **depression** two years previously.

> **"Aha!" More copycat.** Dylan graduated from high school with lifetime membership in the California Scholarship Federation. He went to California State Polytechnic University at Pomona, **the university his brother, Jason, attended**, when he died. Dylan lived in the dorm where Jason lived and learned what he felt he needed to know about the school. After about a year there, Dylan wanted to go to the school **where Justin now was**, the University of California at Los Angeles. University Admissions told him he could not transfer to UCLA, as he had already been accepted into the state university system at Cal Poly, unless he went to a junior college for a year.

So he did. There, he met Vanessa. After the year in junior college, both he and she packed up and moved the four hundred miles to live together so Dylan **could go to UCLA along with brother Justin**.

After about a semester, Vanessa had endured enough of their cramped studio apartment and maybe of Dylan, and moved out. Because she was pregnant with our grandchild, we successfully invited her to live with us, now in Sacramento, for the course of her pregnancy.

Dylan finished his term in Los Angeles, then came back the four hundred miles to our condo, moving in with us and Vanessa in time to share in the birth of their daughter, Brittney.

Because it was apparent to us that Dylan had some very real issues with **anger** and **depression**, and because he was still a student, we found that through Mike's insurance we could get him an appointment to see if a counselor could help him, Vanessa, and our newborn granddaughter.

> **"Aha!" No surprises, please.** Dylan showed up for the appointment. He found an empty room (sans receptionist and without any clue as to how to proceed), saw a door with the counselor's name on it, and entered. He found the counselor and another client in a session. Being told that he had done the wrong thing by opening the door and going in, Dylan bolted and never went back. No counseling this time.

Surprises and Aspies **do not mix. Breach of routine** or expectations can send one into **meltdown** or **flight**.

Now that Dylan had achieved fatherhood but had not completed his education, he decided to go to yet another (the fourth) college, California State University at Chico, which was only about two hours north of us, instead of a day's travel away in Los Angeles. His new family went with him; Dylan and Vanessa, for the sake of their child, or in the interest of meeting the expectations of their families, tried once again to make the relationship work.

> **"Aha!" Flight.** A few months later, Mike and I made a planned visit to their apartment near the university to enjoy a family visit and to catch up with our young granddaughter. Dylan was not home; he had some kind of blowup or meltdown with Vanessa, and simply left.

This again is the **flight** factor. He could not cope, so he just left.

Not long after that, Vanessa and Brittney left the Chico apartment and moved back to the Sacramento area, while Dylan continued with school and with playing rugby in Chico. He was able to come home during holidays and school breaks to share some time with his daughter, visiting for the most part with her at our house.

While at Chico State University, Dylan became romantically involved with another young woman, Aimee. Dylan had earned a bachelor's degree in English, but because Aimee had not yet earned her degree, Dylan chose to stay at the university, enrolling in the master's program. They soon eloped.

By impulsively marrying, an Aspie can simply preempt all the social fuss attending a traditional wedding. By **avoidance**, he did not have to face the social implications of ceremonial unions where skill in introductions and small talk are prerequisites. The social preparation of planning and executing a traditional wedding are overwhelming to an Aspie. So Dylan opted to **sidestep the traditional ceremony**.

We met Aimee and her parents, who gave them a home wedding reception. We thought and hoped that maybe, at last, Dylan could find some happiness and would calm down and accept the social responsibility of a marriage relationship. He did find a summer job painting apartment interiors.

I specifically remember telling Aimee's mother, at the reception, that Dylan had a lot of anger, especially after his brother's passing, but now seemed calmer (crediting her daughter while also giving her a "heads-up").

Not long after marriage, in the fall of 1995, Aimee and Dylan traveled to London, England, where Dylan eventually got a job and took delight in having his photo taken with the statue of poet Lord Byron. Dylan had read everything by the poet and seemed **fixed** in this **special interest**. However, when their student exchange work visa expired after three months, the young couple returned to Northern California.

As Christmas was coming up, and Aimee had not had much chance to get to know her now four-year-old stepdaughter, Brittney, Mike and I gave them, as a present, what we thought would be a "bonding" trip to Disneyland.

> **"Aha!" Inappropriate outbursts.** At the end of the trip, when we picked up the three of them at the airport, I could tell that all was *not* well. Dylan seemed absolutely ready to explode with anger, barely managing to contain it until he finally burst out yelling, in the car, on the way home, "Next time, just give us the money instead!"

Socially inappropriate and unexpected outbursts are another Aspie trait. Communication is incomplete—not related to a reciprocal exchange of parties. Dylan had never picked up on the social clue that even if he would rather have had the money, it was **not acceptable to voice that preference**. We had no idea why he was so mad and opted not to discuss it for fear of escalating tempers.

Then we discovered that the windows of Aimee's car, which was parked in front of our house while they were gone, were broken, and that her radio or speakers had been stolen. Dylan yelled at us that we had to fix her car.

Again, **inappropriate adult behavior**.

> **"Aha!" Difficulty with relationships.** The new couple returned to Chico. We were *not* sensing the development of a supportive marital relationship as Mike and I knew it. We were further disheartened, then overcome with grief and angst, when we got home from work one evening to find Dylan at our home, sitting with his back to the room entry, facing the computer, just kind of staring, obviously in some kind of shock.

> **"Aha!" Self-injury.** Not only that, his face had apparently been beaten. It was swollen, bruised and abraded, with bloodied eyes.

Sinking, the only question I could squeak out was, "What happened?"

"I did it."

No more questions were asked, but we surmised the marriage was over . . . and we were grateful that he had come home.

The **difficulty with relationships** stems from the inability to understand social interaction and is one of the core features and absolute realities of anyone on the autistic spectrum. It is very difficult for an Aspie to maintain an enduring romantic relationship, especially when neither party has a clue as to the communication difficulties of an AS person. The repeated failure of relationships is devastating to an Aspie. It is not uncommon for **self-injurious behavior**, or the ultimate, **suicide**, to follow the hopelessness brought on by romantic failures.

> **"Aha!" Depression without help.** We took Dylan under our wing for a few weeks, as his face healed, but his depression was increasing. We guessed that the university master's program was over too. He continued to work out at a gym, twice a day, every day. We saw this as a good sign, knowing that physical exercise is therapy for depression.
>
> With his depression and anger so apparent, and because of our past experience with Jason and fearing the worst, I tried frantically to find a psychiatrist to help Dylan, either with medication or with *whatever would work*. I pursued everything I could to avert the dreaded consequence . . . .
>
> The first twenty-two calls did not produce results because the only qualifying question the person answering the phone asked me was, does he have insurance? My answer was "No." No insurance, no help.

> Since Dylan was through schooling and in his midtwenties, he did not qualify for coverage under Mike's insurance policy.
>
> Everyone thought it was strange that I, mother to an *adult* person, would be seeking the help. (Why couldn't he do it himself?)

We didn't know it at that time, but now know that an Aspie takes **little social initiative**, especially for "help." Recognizing the need for help and getting assistance is a complex social process whereby one must first name the "problem," then figure out what to do, where to go and to whom to talk. All complex social functions. He very likely **would not even try to communicate his issues to an appropriate agency or person**. As for my involvement, I only did what I deemed necessary for me to do regardless of our son's (adult) age.

Call 23 found me a psychiatrist near our home who would see Dylan if I brought $100 to his office on the mornings of the appointments. I agreed, and, remembering my previous failure in getting Dylan connected with a counselor, asked the appointment maker for very specific instructions to relay to Dylan about what he could expect and how he should proceed to prevent him from bolting again.

As with the previously aborted counseling appointment, **knowing what to expect** ahead of time is very important to an Aspie. It is **difficult to change focus** or **understand spontaneously** what to do when a social situation is unexpected.

Dylan went to his first psychiatric appointment. All I learned from Dylan after that visit was that the doctor would not prescribe medication without further analysis of Dylan's situation or condition. OK. A subsequent appointment was made for the following week.

After about three weeks, with his face nearly healed, Dylan moved out of our house to live with other rugby players from Chico in Walnut Creek, which by car is at least an hour and a half away. We loaned him a vehicle, and he was able to make it back to his second appointment with the psychiatrist a week later. So far, so good, but still no medication. I could hardly physically let go of his arm so he could drive back to his new home, as I feared I might never see him alive again.

The next week I again gladly took the "C-note" to the doctor's office, assuming that Dylan would drive up to Sacramento for his next appointment as he had done the week before. Instead, began what I now refer to as the most difficult day of my life.

Question: So what is more difficult than our previous experience of hearing that our firstborn chose to die by train? Answer: Knowing that another son's life is in crisis and that *whatever little thing* you do or say either can cause or avert the ultimate consequence . . . .

The phone call; it was an obviously upset Dylan who flatly, angrily stated that he "was fucking going to kill somebody today." Stunned, I remember barely stammering out, "Who do you have in mind"? Answer: "Myself."

All I could think to do was to plead with him to call a suicide prevention line. I then called suicide prevention myself. They asked me if Dylan had a gun. I said I didn't think so. She said, "Go there, then call suicide prevention again when you get there. Go there."

Atypically, no argument from me this time. I hurriedly called his psychiatrist, quickly mentioned the unfolding situation, and asked him to call Dylan immediately. He agreed to do so then asked that I call him back later.

Straightaway I called Mike at work then picked him up, and we drove, shaken to our cores and hardly breathing, while tension, responsibility, fear, and desperation all concomitantly flooded our senses.

I was not going to lose this child too! All we had was a piece of paper with directions as to how to get to his address and an hour and a half of roadway between us and where we might find him, hopefully alive.

We found the address, a two-story house on a residential street. Ominously, the front screen door was hanging askew by one hinge only. We knew Dylan's anger and the previous throwing of the saucepan, and it took no imagination to guess how the door got broken.

All was quiet except for our insistent knocking on the door . . . *More* knocking, no answer . . . . I couldn't help myself and just yelled, **"Dylan!"**

Oh my god, oh my god, his angry yell back—"What?"—came from upstairs. *We were in time!*

But it wasn't over. Suicide prevention, which we now called from Dylan's, told us to bring him to a Contra Costa County facility to be evaluated. We were thankful to be able to get some help. The half-hour drive up the freeway was almost as tense as our drive to Walnut Creek, as I saw, considering Dylan's barely controlled rage, a real possibility that he would open the car's backseat door and jump out onto the freeway . . . .

(Apparently the psychiatrist from Sacramento had called Dylan, as I requested. All Dylan had to say about that was that he "hated" him.)

After sitting silently for what seemed like about two hours, waiting among a whole crowd of more visibly needy persons, we, these three adults with no apparent disabilities, handicaps, or medical crises, were called to the second floor.

Once there, we had to ring a bell and announce ourselves. It dawned on me that this is a locked "Psych" ward. With visions of Electro Convulsive Therapy, padded rooms, and forced sedative injections from my prior employment as a Psychiatric Technician in a locked mental hospital, I wondered if we had done the right thing or if we had made matters worse.

Dylan was let into the facility with the stipulation that in this place he would not be allowed to hurt himself or anyone else. He was asked a few questions about payment and his marital status. With obvious recoil, and an ironic snort, Dylan flatly and quickly said, "Divorced." First Vanessa, now Aimee. Gone.

After disappearing with Dylan for about twenty minutes, a "social worker" came to talk to us. Not only did he seem miffed that we as parents were there, as Dylan was an "adult," he shared with us that he could have locked Dylan up but thought that would not be the best thing to do. (We agreed.) He then gave Dylan his business card and said that Dylan could call him anytime. I can tell you that never happened. That guy was just one more "idiot" to Dylan.

In the elevator down, Dylan accused us of "lying" to him. Not being sure of his meaning, I didn't say anything in hopes that the entire circumstance could now at least be diffused.

We took him back to his residence, then reluctantly left, as we heard what sounded like crashing pots or pans . . . .

I did call the psychiatrist when Mike and I returned home. Of course, he could not breach confidentiality by talking with me about what Dylan had told him, but I got hints from the doctor that perhaps Dylan's threat of suicide was a maneuver to get something from us (manipulation).

Even though for several years we could see that Dylan was nearly indigent, though a college graduate, we made sure not to give financial assistance so as not to be enablers. Now, in the Aspie context, we can see that Dylan never, even in his neediness, insinuated or asked for anything! Our concerns about enabling were unfounded and the psychiatrist's hints to us that Dylan was trying to "work" us were no doubt based on neurotypical analysis. AS persons, unlike NTs, do not have the subtle but complex social skills needed to direct or otherwise control the behavior of others. An Aspie is not likely to be aware of social pressure as bargaining ante. He is **not manipulative**.

Shortly thereafter, Dylan returned to temporarily stay with us in Sacramento. We were happy to "reparent," as it were, if we could give him support without having him become dependent on us. And he continued to work out at a nearby gym regularly, twice a day.

> **"Aha!" Workaholic.** During those few weeks, Dylan worked for us, painting the interior and refurbishing an outside wooden fence. I remember specifically noting that he worked very carefully and reliably, and that was a very positive aspect about him. At that time we said to ourselves that even though he does not follow the path of our expectations, or any identifiable path for that matter, he at least had role modeled a very strong work ethic.

Post-Aspiedom realization, I now see his quality of work, attention to detail, and his dependability less as role modeling, less as ethic, and more as **what Aspies do to maintain a sense of order and predictability in their lives**.

> **"Aha!" Familial disconnect.** Dylan had several visits with his daughter, who lived about twenty miles away from us, but never seemed to connect with her in the expected father role where he would find a way to share in her life in a permanent way. (Not that any of us—Brittney's mom, Mike, or I—encouraged him to do so, knowing his apparent emotional difficulties, and Brittney's apparent well-being with her mom.) Having my own interest in getting to see my granddaughter, I accompanied him to a court custody hearing. Vanessa's arrival was delayed, and by default, Dylan was awarded shared custody. We never pressed him to actually share time of custody, thinking only of the best interest of Brittney; nor did he press the matter.

Family is the most basic social unit in which NT adults fill the roles of male and female leadership, providing modeling and socialization for their children. But an Aspie, even though he may beget children, is barely socialized himself and the role of parental leadership may not be fully grasped. It is **difficult for an AS person to lead**, taking **responsibility** for a family. This is especially true if he isn't aware of his presence in Aspiedom and has therefore not learned any social accommodation thereof.

After a few weeks, Dylan moved briefly to Las Vegas, where he slept in his car. He then returned to the Los Angeles area. He had a hard time getting a job, but his brother, Justin, came through, finding him work first as a bouncer, then as a bartender at the same club where Justin worked in Hollywood. Dylan lived alone in a seedy, crime-prone hotel (the desk clerk was shot while Dylan resided there).

After a couple of years there, with no phone and very little contact with us, he decided to do what he knew his brothers, Mike, and I had done before he was even born—take a tour of the country. Now, at thirty years old, he packed up his pickup truck, and with a gas credit card donated by Mike and I, and his national gym membership, took off to visit sites that interested him, particularly the homes of favorite authors he knew from his ravenous reading, especially sites involving horror. He showered at the fitness clubs and slept in his pickup truck in the gym parking lots.

He wanted to visit Midland-Odessa, Texas, the setting for *Friday Nights Lights*. He wanted to see the house in Holcomb, Kansas, where the quadruple murders of the Clutter family occurred and which Truman Capote had documented in his book *In Cold Blood*. He wanted to get close to the home of horror novelist Stephen King, in Maine, the home of Ernest Hemingway in Key West, Florida, and the home of J.D. Salinger in Cornish, New Hampshire. And he did—all of them.

His **fascination** with true crime, **blood and guts**, and horror continued, but we finally were feeling that he was "on his path" when he made a decision to head off on an adventure such as this. He kept a journal, but did not publish anything that we were aware of. He clearly maintained his interest in the language, as well as in the persons who wrote stories that interested him.

As reading is a solitary activity where social participation is not required, Aspies often are **avid readers (hyperlexia)**. It is also hypothesized that in fiction, the written word tells how characters feel, ergo there is no need to guess how someone feels or thinks as is required in real time with real people in actual social encounters.

During this cross-country trip he also visited New Orleans (**as he knew, we and his brothers had done** before he was born) and found something there compelling enough to make him to want to move there, isolating himself from his family, but finding a lot of action happening all about him, if not because of him.

He secured a bartending job on Bourbon Street in the French Quarter, and lives in New Orleans today. He has had several different bartending jobs and two housing moves within "The Quarter." He still tends bar, though he prefers, incongruously, "not to talk to the customers."

Dylan returned home to California a couple of times for Christmas and Thanksgiving family get-togethers, and when he was forced to leave New Orleans a week and a half after hurricane Katrina. Each time during the holiday reunions when he and Justin were both present, there would be a fight of some kind. One time Dylan left our house for a few hours; one time Justin left, flying directly back to Los Angeles to avoid Dylan. I'm sure Justin could write his own book on the subject of his disconcerting relationship with his brother.

After Katrina, Dylan's visit home was for about a week. What is particularly memorable about the visit is that at the age of thirty-six, this was his last time home as a *nonidentified Aspie*.

We wondered so many times why this bright, artistically talented young man just could not get employment suitable to his interests and to his university degree in English. We couldn't fathom why he did not seem interested in a professional career, an art career, or any career where there was advancement opportunity, benefits, and financial security! We didn't "get" Dylan's apparent lack of fatherly connection to his daughter.

On the first anniversary of Hurricane Katrina, I heard the television reporters giving their accounts of having been stationed there one year previous, during the big storm. One well-recognized CNN reporter stood just outside the French Quarter club where Dylan was working, but never came in to talk to Dylan, or anyone else for that matter, about their personal experience of working in New Orleans or staying on site during the hurricane.

So we had all kinds of newspaper and television news stories and accounts from those who visited New Orleans as reporters; but we heard not one written, first-person account of anyone who lived in New Orleans, had refused to leave during Hurricane Katrina, did not need rescuing, did not loot, and had endured the whole catastrophe as well as the aftermath. To judge by television reports alone, no one had done that.

The only way those of us who live outside of New Orleans could learn of the big storm in the "Big Easy" was from reporters who went there solely for the storm, who had protection and secure provisions, and who had no personal investment in the storm's impact.

Well, Dylan was there. He had the whole experience, hunkered down securing the club where he worked, eating the previously frozen food that was thawing due to the lack of electricity, drinking the club's available bottled water, behaving himself and doing without a shower. He can write. Why did he not use the opportunity to write his story? His dad, the primary role model, would have done exactly that. We could have had that first-person account.

> **"Aha!" Fearlessness.** Though it might have seemed rash not to leave New Orleans during Katrina, the Aspie element of irrational daring characterizes Dylan.

> **"Aha!" Failure to role model.** We could not at first figure out why Dylan did not take this marvelous opportunity to create a first-person account and sell a book, like his father would have done. All his life, he had seen his dad take notes and write stories for publication. With Dylan's formal education in English, his writing history (the book of poems), his awards ("Promising Author"), and his constant need for money, it just did not make sense that he would not capitalize on Hurricane Katrina and write that first-person account.

If he had modeled Mike, he would have captured on paper the sounds of terrorizing winds, the thrill of hiding, waiting it out, and surviving the destruction. He would have written about witnessing the breakdown of law and the city being taken over by gun-wielding National Guard soldiers. He could have shared the smells of decay and waste in the aftermath. His report could have been a unique account of one who was an emotionally invested resident and stayed the course of Hurricane Katrina.

Now we know why, from two Aspie-aware perspectives, why he did not pursue that account. First, AS persons **do not role model** (see **POSTSCRIPT**). Identification with the parent of the same gender is the lead psychosocial process involved in neurotypical growing up, ergo, socialization. But when one is an Aspie, the social context or "model" is not incorporated. He could not "see" his adult self in the role of his father.

Second, self-marketing, recognizing and making the most of an opportunity, is a complex function rooted in contextual social importance, and involves nuanced **executive functions**. It demands **drawing a conclusion, grasping the main idea**, then **initiating** and **sustaining behavior** to reach a goal. It demands **planning, prioritizing, sequencing, and realizing the social impact of an activity**. These are overwhelming and alien processes to an Aspie.

This **absence of role modeling** (and book writing) as related to the first anniversary of Hurricane Katrina was my last reminiscence of Dylan's behavioral oddities before reading the two words, "Asperger's Syndrome" and my resulting epiphany. It is my last **"Aha!"**

From that time forward, I've had my answer to the enigmas of rearing Dylan. *At last,* his behavioral anomalies have their name, and it is Asperger's Syndrome. *At last,* my curiosity has been satisfied. *At last,* after all those years of not having a clue to appropriately understand and parent my own son, I "get" it . . . .

DYLAN
"Ahhh!"

"There's a divinity that shapes our ends,
Rough hew them how we will."

—*Hamlet*

"Aha!" + "Aha!" + "Aha!" = "Ahhh," relief. At least for me. Right along, as I read more and more about Aspiedom, I expressed to Mike the Dylan/Aspie trait matches. He agreed with my remembrances and "Aha!" pairings, but often played the devil's advocate, suggesting that there might be other answers. So even though for the most part he has come to accept Dylan in Aspiedom, he remains open to supplementary explanations.

What has always been clear to both of us, however, was that Dylan's personality dissonance and familial asymmetry begged *some* explanation. His behavioral traits and talents were too clearly unique to fit into the sociological context of our family. His artistic talent and aggressive behaviors seemed particularly incongruous. We knew *something* was going on with him but were clueless as to *what that something was*. Consequently, we grabbed onto any possible explanation that would account for his disparateness.

Ironically, we never considered that there might be a genetic component! Instead, we seized environmental hypotheses to illuminate our puzzle and to help us decipher our situation. In order of magnitude, here are the factors we settled on for accountability (the first thirty-six years), *prior* to grasping the essence of Asperger's Syndrome:

Conception. Dylan was conceived through a double dose of spermicide. That's right, through vaginal foam prophylactic. We knew it was time for ovulation and had nothing against bearing another child, except that we were altruistic proponents of the ZPG (Zero Population Growth) movement popular in the hippie culture of 1970. We already had borne our allotted two self-replacement children. Hence, we used a pregnancy preventative, double dosing to ensure (so we assumed) effectiveness.

Electroshock. Dylan was about seven weeks gestation, and I was feeling justified and happy, despite the outside ZPG influence, that this baby was "meant to be." (And as I pen these biographical pages, the notion of "meant to be" has found its full expression.) We were camping in an area where there was an electric fence, with the "juice" turned up (for sheep, I think). Our then almost four-year-old Jason somehow touched the fence and with the electricity coursing through him, became paralyzed. He could not let go of the fence and just screamed. Thankfully, I had been witness to a similar situation some years earlier with a screaming child being "frozen" to a pinball machine. In that scenario, I saw a large man quickly grab the boy away, concomitantly forcing a break in the electric circuit, absorbing the jolt with his larger body and releasing the child. So as any parent would do, I lunged for my child, likewise absorbing the electricity with my larger body and pulled my child to safety. But being that I was pregnant, embryonic Dylan surely took on the electric shock as well. I frequently remembered back to that incident as a possible explanation for Dylan's singularity.

Omission. Because Dylan began assisted walking early, at six months, he crawled very little. I later learned that infant crawling was vital to normal brain development and that children who did not crawl or did not crawl enough could have developmental issues. At the time I learned of this, therapists were treating children who didn't crawl by physically manipulating their arms and legs to replicate the cross-lateral movement thought to activate the development of nerve pathways between the brain's two hemispheres. Did the fact that Dylan omitted crawling alter his brain's development, resulting in our witnessed behavioral curiosities?

Addition. Five years before Dylan was born, I had read about the concept of a "supermale," a male child born with an extra Y-chromosome that hypothetically explained aggressiveness. Remembering and matching that hypothesis to Dylan's behavior, I mused that maybe Dylan had that extra Y-chromosome. Perhaps.

Rough-hewn as it seems, we now have our AS epiphany, and at last have a comprehensive denouement to our Dylan dilemmas. His/the family's thirty-six-year saga finally makes sense in the Asperger's Syndrome context. We do breathe that sigh of relief.

About informing Dylan, then. The next step had to be to bring Asperger's Syndrome to the attention of this improbably strong, young man, who from the very beginning had overcome sperm assassins and embryo tazing just to get here.

At first, the imperative was clear to contact him *now*, as soon as possible. For years we had known Dylan's volatility and could only hope that he would "mature" out of it. In the meantime, not confident about the maturity part, we were concerned that it would be only a matter of time before he was in social, emotional, or legal trouble.

Certainly, the Asperger's Syndrome answer would bring him, as well as us, some relief. That is, if he could immediately see and accept the probability. Maybe just knowing, just having a name and a concept, would put the puzzle pieces of his life into order. Maybe knowledge would lessen his angst, frustration, and volatility; and help him understand why relating to others personally and in the workplace is difficult for him. Why his anger is often in his way. Without this information to help his identity, he seemed but one paycheck away from being homeless or another failed romance away from being hopeless.

However, I alternatively recognized that my declaration of Asperger's Syndrome to Dylan might be a cause for contention or further angst. Labels are only helpful in the right context.

But I did not deliberate for long and quickly decided to take the risk of awakening Dylan's agitation, in the event that something troublesome would happen *before* I did *everything I could* to inform him and allay trouble. We would, of course, give him emotional support.

> Tuesday, 4/10
>
> Dear Dylan,
>
> Enclosed, please find a few pages about Asperger's Syndrome. I pass them along to you with the hope that if you find an identity here, you will also find some relief.
>
> It's important to me that you know I am here to support you and love you.
>
> I'll do everything in my power to get you a professional diagnosis, if that is what you want.
>
> Please call us when you get this mail.
>
> In the meantime, if you are wanting to confer with your County health services, you can "walk in" after 8:30 am to the Charter-Pontchartrain facility on Elysian Fields. Payment is on a "sliding scale," based on ability to pay. I would encourage you to start there with a social worker,

then a doctor, especially if you feel anxious or depressed. They will give you a questionnaire to fill out, checking off symptoms.

Always know we care — please keep in touch.

Love,
Marti & Mike

Letter to Dylan

"Dear Dylan,

Enclosed, please find a few pages about Asperger's Syndrome.

I pass them along to you with the hope that if you find an identity here, you will also find some relief.

It is important to me that you know I am here to support you and love you. I'll do everything in my power to get you a professional diagnosis, if that is what you want.

Please call us when you get this mail.

In the meantime, if you want to confer with your county health services, you can "walk in" after 8:30 am to the Charter-Pontchartrain facility on Elyssian Fields. Payment is on a "sliding scale," based on ability to pay.

I encourage you to start there with a social worker, then a doctor, especially if you feel anxious or depressed. They will give you a questionnaire to fill out, checking off symptoms.

Always know we care. Please keep in touch. Love, Marti and Mike"

On Formal Diagnosis

At this juncture, I had not yet shifted my own perspective beyond the medical paradigm of Asperger's Syndrome and thought Dylan needed a formal diagnosis. And after a phone conversation with him, I knew he preferred the same.

In my search for the appropriate diagnostic professional, I received the following good advice via e-mail from Jim Sinclair, autistic adult, rehabilitation counselor, and coordinator of Autism Network International:

> "Adults with Asperger's Syndrome often have a hard time finding a professional diagnosis. Diagnosis is generally made by a clinical psychologist, neuropsychologist, or psychiatrist. If you happen to live near a major autism research and treatment center, that would be a place to start... Be sure to hold out until you find a clinician who's actually experienced at evaluating and diagnosing adults with AS. Clinicians who are only experienced with autistic children, or with nonverbal autistic people, are woefully inadequate at recognizing Asperger's Syndrome in adults."[1]

So I did start with a major autism research and treatment center:
The MIND Institute, University of California, Davis:
"He's *how* old?"
"Thirty-six."
Rejection 1 (Children only)

Psychoneuroplasticity Center (PNP), Lewisville, Texas: By phone, "The cost of the 'work up' is about $7,000." Plus lodging, airfare, time away from work.

I wrote a letter asking for some kind of grant or scholarship for adults. **Rejection 2** (They did not reply.)

Several private psychiatrists listed by various Asperger's Syndrome associations: "Does he have insurance?" (I knew this game from my previous efforts.)
"No."
Rejection 3, etc., etc., etc.

I also looked online for active research studies involving autism and inquired whether Dylan or the whole family could volunteer. *All of them* required a "formal diagnosis." So **rejection** from them as well.

Well, guess what. My efforts at securing any such thing were thwarted so many times that I came to see that not only were there no qualified persons available to "diagnose" Dylan, there was really no need to do so. He is who he is, and always has been, *regardless* of not having a formal diagnosis.

What was I or he to do with a diagnosis? We were not looking for excuses, sympathy, or services. We sought only awareness, self-understanding and acknowledgement. The "Ahhh!" factor.

Furthermore, in my continuing research, I was finding that most adult Aspies have either self-identified, or had someone bring the possibility to their attention, and then upon reading the AS traits, found recognition. I later learned that in fact there *are no* definitive, objective criteria that can identify Asperger's Syndrome. Any professional diagnosis would depend on my and Dylan's accounts of his personal history as well as their observations and subjectivity.

Until science provides a definitive test that can positively, irrevocably register anyone's presence in *or* out of Aspiedom, I stand firm. Based on the information from my research and personal knowledge of Dylan's history, the most likely explanation of Dylan's stellar bumptiousness is indeed his presence in that mysterious, fascinating land of Aspiedom.

The bottom line: One psychiatrist in New Orleans (where Dylan lives) did respond to my e-mail with his office phone number. When I called, he was kind enough—because Dylan did not have insurance or other financial means to secure a private physician—to refer me (for Dylan) to a clinic in the city. Access was available with a sliding scale payment program.

However, to take advantage of a government program (for the uninsured and medically indigent), the prospective patient or client must *ask for help himself*. This premise assumes neurotypical adult socialization and, though understandable, certainly leaves out anyone, such as an Aspie, who is not inclined to ask for help. Dylan would need to take the initiative to set up his own case, which he did manage by following my advice outlined in the letter above.

Dylan saw a physician at the clinic, but she would not diagnose Asperger's Syndrome at that time. (Dr.: "What makes you think you have Asperger's Syndrome?" Dylan: "My mom.") The doctor *did* formally diagnose Dylan with Bipolar Disorder, Depression, and Alcoholism. She prescribed medication. These three diagnoses are all common attendees to AS. At this time, because there is only a minimal awareness of AS *adults*, it is inconsequential, except for personal edification, to seek diagnosis. We, in this culture, provide very little special education, government assistance, or organized support for this unique adult population. However, we are gradually waking up to the need. The chapter "LOOKING FORWARD" details some programs.

Though Dylan is without a formal Asperger's Syndrome diagnosis, in his new awareness of AS he is gaining understanding of the profile of Aspiedom. He has expressed relief. "I'm glad it's Asperger's, I thought I was just an ass."

Differential profiles: To clarify the difference between an adult in NT land and one in Aspiedom, I offer a comparison of the (socialized) NT profile with Dylan's de facto adult profile.

NT adult profile (Lives by the social rules; *is socialized.*)
- Career—Applies his education, talent, and interests; expands his prospects for a productive, meaningful life. Takes proactive interest in self-promotion to increase his level of success.
- Civics—Takes an interest in and affiliates in his community and participates in government, demonstrated by keeping informed, voting, and filing a tax return.
- Well-being—Seeks support from physician, dentist, optometrist.
- Insurance—Protects himself by securing medical and appropriate liability insurance.
- Identification—Maintains current identification, such as a driver's license, photo ID, or passport.
- Fiscal responsibility—Establishes bank accounts and credit for fiscal grounding.
- Family and friends—Establishes friendships and a permanent bonding with another adult, begets and rears children, makes a home and supports a family and self as a private/independent unit.
- Eye on the future—Plans and invests appropriately now so that he will not be destitute in the future.

This profile translates into a real-time adult life with security, direction, connection, and purpose.

Aspiedom (Dylan's) adult profile: (What social rules? If the rules are not seen as logical, they are out. "I make my own rules." [Dylan, 2008])
- Job—Has a job and is a focused, dependable worker. However, he is underemployed. His interests, intelligence, and talents are not used in developing work or career. He has no employment "benefits."
- Talent—Has no desire or idea as to how to market himself.
- Civics—Usually votes, or at least "thinks about it," but may not file a tax return.
- Well-being—Physician, no. Dentist, no. Optometrist, no. Gym workouts, yes.
- Insurance—What for and with what money?
- Identification—Has an expired driver's license and a current (for now) passport.
- Fiscal responsibility—No bank account, no credit and may still have outstanding loans.
- Family and friends—Has parented a child, but has not established the socially expected permanent parent-child bonding. Emotional attachment to his child is skewed, and the concept of being a role model is, at best, academic. He does note that "mysteriously though, she loves me." Friends are primarily the people with whom he works.
- Eye on future—This adult in Aspiedom is still trying to fit into the present. What's the big deal about the future?

This profile adds up to a precarious, unsupported independent life. It is further complicated by the attending conditions of depression, aggression, and alcohol overuse.

"Is he lazy?" "Does he have character flaws?" "Is he retarded?" "What's wrong with him?" "Why can't he just be an ordinary adult?" Understandably, one might ask these questions when first assessing the above profile. The answers are, "No." "No." "No," and "Nothing is wrong with him, and he is *not* and never will be an ordinary adult."

Mike and I have found the name for our enigmas, accept our findings, and value them for what they are. We have pressed the reset button, and have newly begun to appreciate Dylan for the neuroexceptional person he is . . . .

WHAT IS IT?

"O, there has been much throwing about of brains."
—Hamlet

Concept, Nomenclature, Spectrum, Syndrome
Asperger's Syndrome is a concept: Dysfunction. Disability. Disease. Difference. Debility. Affliction. Gift. Mental Illness. Brain abnormality. Brain disorder. Neurobiological disorder. Neurobehavioral condition. Genetic disease. Neurological disorder. Psychiatric disorder. Developmental disorder. Serious psychological illness. Positive identity, not a disability. Alternative way of being. Mental health condition. Neurodevelopmental disorder in the Autism Spectrum. Neuroexceptional condition. Autism lite. Mental health illness!

Honest! Throughout my research, I read and recorded, with each word or phrase from a separate source, all of the above descriptors for the *same condition*. The value of noting them here is to demonstrate the difficulty of understanding or expressing the essence of Asperger's Syndrome.

However, the AS concept is articulated by an Aspie himself, Vernon Smith, Nobel Laureate in economic sciences, who acknowledges that the syndrome has deficiencies, but "may actually have some selective advantages..."[1] For our purposes here, we'll agree with him and humbly add that these deficiencies and advantages are neurologically based, stable, and lifelong.

Asperger's Syndrome is nomenclature: Autism Spectrum Disorder or Asperger's Syndrome Disorder (**ASD**). Asperger's Syndrome (**AS**). Asperger Syndrome (also **AS**). Aspergers. Asperger Autism. High-Functioning Autism (**HFA**). Pervasive Developmental Disorder, Not Otherwise Specified (**PDD-NOS**).

Basically, we are talking about the same condition using all of the above terms. There is a difference between **HFA** and **AS**, but it applies primarily when a person is being formally diagnosed. In **HFA**, language is not developed by the age of two. In **AS**, language is developed by the age of two. A person who is diagnosed (especially as a child) as **HFA** is considered "autistic" and often will qualify for social services or special education. One who is diagnosed with **AS** often is not as readily accepted as "autistic" and therefore may not be eligible for the same services as an **HFA** person. As an adult, the difference in age of language acquisition is not discernible, and therefore is not relevant for our discussion. High-Functioning Autism and Asperger's Syndrome are regarded here as a single entity.

PDD-NOS is a general category to denote that one *is* on the autistic spectrum. A professional may diagnose **PDD-NOS**, declining to make or preliminary to making the **HFA/AS**, or other distinction. Often, on rediagnosis, **PDD-NOS** is refined to an **AS** diagnosis.

In discussions about the autistic spectrum and pervasive developmental disorders, Rett's Syndrome and Childhood Disintegrative Disorder are often mentioned because they share several signs with autism, but are thought to have unrelated causes. They are classified as separate from AS, but do bear some relevance to our discussion of spectrum.

Additional research certainly will draw more important lines of distinction for these designations, and no doubt also will identify and provide boundaries for subcategories of Asperger's Syndrome. Scientific sifting may discover differing etiologies or may establish other criteria necessary to delineate one concept or fraction of concept from the others.

Asperger's Syndrome is on a spectrum: Dr. Lorna Wing, a British MD and researcher, in 1991 popularized the term "Asperger's Syndrome." She and her colleague, clinical psychologist Judith Gould, PhD, pioneered the concept of the "autistic spectrum." This autistic (or autism) spectrum is the fundamental operative concept for our discussion of Asperger's Syndrome. No matter what one calls the condition, it is part of a singular concept of *autism that manifests on a spectrum*. And no matter where one lies on that spectrum, the core identifying features will be the same.

In discussing AS, it is helpful to divide the spectrum into two aspects: classic autism on one side, and Asperger's Syndrome on the other. The divide between classic autism and AS is at the point where *language* is manifest, *and* where average or above cognitive development can be accurately gauged. An Aspie presents with language (sometimes verbosity), and most often with considerable cognitive ability.

Now, the question becomes, what defines the terminus at the end of the spectrum? Where does AS end and NT begin? Does Aspiedom fade gradually into Neurotypical Land? Is the threshold arbitrary, or is there a clear division between Aspiedom and the terrain of NTs?

It would be very satisfying academically to intersect a vertical line across our spectrum line that would say autism, including AS, is on one side of that line and neurotypicity continues to the other side.

For now, however, we have no such reckoning. We just get there in a linguistic concept, without knowing exactly where the line of demarcation is.

And the reason we don't know where the AS/NT line is drawn is we do not have a way to definitively, scientifically, objectively recognize that a line even exists. "Unfortunately, there are no specific genetic or biological markers that accurately identify a person as being on this autism spectrum," writes Marylin Smith Carsley in the *Westmount Examiner*.[2]

Therefore, there simply is no hard claim to either side of the dividing line between Aspiedom and Neurotypical Land. There is no blood test, no X-ray, no MRI, EEG, neuroSPECT scan, no swab, no smear, nor any form of poking or squeezing or inserting that can assuage our need for such circumscription. IQ tests can be administered; general state of health can be evaluated. Brain scans are useful research tools that show undefined atypical activity. But we are right back to subjective, observable behaviors for Asperger's identification. We'll have to leave the question of provable parameters to expanded scientific investigation.

So though it is unclear as to exactly where on the autistic spectrum Asperger's Syndrome abuts neurotypicity, this spectrum is nonetheless *the* umbrella postulate that allows us to discuss Asperger's Syndrome as an entity.

Asperger's is a *syndrome*: Though we have only the subjective means of observation and personal history to identify it, we do have many consistent hints and hallmarks to confirm the Aspie identity. It is this "set" or *collection of behavioral markers consistently occurring together* that are the gestalt of Asperger's Syndrome.

Discovery of Asperger's Syndrome Essence
Formal, Psychiatric Diagnosis

What are those hallmarks? In professional parlance, those behavioral markers are called "symptoms." So for starters, I give you three standard criteria by which a *formal, medical diagnosis* of Asperger's Syndrome is made.

Diagnostic Criteria For 299.80 Asperger's Disorder
Diagnostic and Statistical Manual of Mental Disorders
(DSM IV), American Psychiatric Association 1994

I. Qualitative impairment in social interaction, as manifested by at least two of the following:
   A. marked impairments in the use of multiple nonverbal behaviors such as eye-to-eye gaze, facial expression, body postures, and gestures to regulate social interaction
   B. failure to develop peer relationships appropriate to developmental level
   C. a lack of spontaneous seeking to share enjoyment, interests, or achievements with other people (e.g. by a lack of showing, bringing, or pointing out objects of interest to other people)
   D. lack of social or emotional reciprocity

II. Restricted repetitive and stereotyped patterns of behavior, interests, and activities, as manifested by at least one of the following:
   A. encompassing preoccupation with one or more stereotyped and restricted patterns of interest that is abnormal either in intensity or focus
   B. apparently inflexible adherence to specific, nonfunctional routines or rituals
   C. stereotyped and repetitive motor mannerisms (e.g., hand or finger flapping or twisting, or complex whole-body movements)
   D. persistent preoccupation with parts of objects

III. The disturbance causes clinically significant impairment in social, occupational, or other important areas of functioning

IV. There is no clinically significant general delay in language (e.g., single words used by age 2 years, communicative phrases used by age 3 years)

V. There is no clinically significant delay in cognitive development or in the development of age-appropriate self-help skills, adaptive behavior (other than social interaction), and curiosity about the environment in childhood

VI. Criteria are not met for another specific Pervasive Developmental Disorder or Schizophrenia

---

Caveat: As this book goes to press, the American Psychiatric Association has proposed that the diagnosis of "Asperger's Disorder" be folded into the general category of "Autism Spectrum Disorder." Final semantic determination will be published in the DSM-5, May 2013. Remember, *whatever the linguistic gymnastics, the condition itself remains unchanged.* (see **LOOKING FORWARD**)

Gillberg's Criteria for Asperger's Disorder
The Biology of the Autistic Syndromes by Christopher Gillberg, Mary Coleman 2nd Edition Cambridge University Press 1992

1. Severe impairment in reciprocal social interaction
(at least two of the following)
    (a) inability to interact with peers
    (b) lack of desire to interact with peers
    (c) lack of appreciation of social cues
    (d) socially and emotionally inappropriate behavior
2. All-absorbing narrow interest
(at least one of the following)
    (a) exclusion of other activities

(b) repetitive adherence
   (c) more rote than meaning
3. Imposition of routines and interests
(at least one of the following)
   (a) on self, in aspects of life
   (b) on others
4. Speech and language problems
(at least three of the following)
   (a) delayed development
   (b) superficially perfect expressive language
   (c) formal, pedantic language
   (d) odd prosody, peculiar voice characteristics
   (e) impairment of comprehension including misinterpretations of literal/implied meanings
5. Nonverbal communication problems
(at least one of the following)
   (a) limited use of gestures
   (b) clumsy/gauche body language
   (c) limited facial expression
   (d) inappropriate expression
   (e) peculiar, stiff gaze
6. Motor clumsiness: poor performance on neurodevelopmental examination

(All six criteria must be met for confirmation of diagnosis.)

Pervasive Developmental Disorders
F84.5 Asperger's syndrome
ICD-10 Classification of Mental and Behavioural Disorders, World Health Organization, Geneva, 1992

A disorder of uncertain nosological validity, characterized by the same kind of qualitative abnormalities of reciprocal social interaction that typify autism, together with a restricted, stereotyped, repetitive repertoire of interests and activities. The disorder differs from autism primarily in that there is no general delay or retardation in language or in cognitive development. Most individuals are of normal general intelligence but it is common for them to be markedly clumsy; the condition occurs predominantly in boys (in a ratio of about eight boys to one girl). It seems highly likely that at least some cases represent mild varieties of autism, but it is uncertain whether or not that is so for all. There is a strong tendency for the abnormalities to persist into adolescence and adult life and it seems that they represent individual characteristics that are not greatly affected by environmental influence. Psychotic episodes occasionally occur in early adult life.

Diagnostic guidelines
Diagnosis is based on the combination of a lack of any clinically significant general delay in language or cognitive development plus, as with autism, the presence of qualitative deficiencies in reciprocal social interaction and restricted, repetitive, stereotyped patterns of behaviour, interests, and activities. There may or may not be problems in communication similar to those associated with autism, but significant language retardation would rule out the diagnosis.

Includes:
- autistic psychopathy
- schizoid disorder of childhood

Excludes:
- anankastic personality disorder (F60.5)
- attachment disorders of childhood (F94.1, F94.2)
- obsessive-compulsive disorder (F42.-)
- schizotypal disorder (F21)
- simple schizophrenia (F20.6)

The above formal criteria draw a convoluted outline around our syndrome so that professionals can, in the absence of hard scientific criteria, offer a diagnosis. They can tell us what AS is by identifying symptoms.

Informal, Nonmedical Identification

However, if we look at AS as a *neurologic* or "brain" state, instead of a *medical* anomaly, we can view Aspiedom from a whole different perspective. We won't even need to talk about "symptoms" and "diagnoses" that need "cures." Those terms belong to medicine.

Instead, we can use neutral words like "traits," "characteristics," "features," "qualities," "attributes," and "behavioral markers." Voila! We can take identification out of the medical lexicon and into user-friendly, personable dialog. We won't even have to think that because someone does not fit the norm he should be cast aside as having something "wrong" with him that necessitates a "cure" to make him "normal."

Accordingly and collectively, we can transpose our perception by allowing the emotional affluence found in acceptance. We can welcome diversity and begin to see what this new paradigm offers. We can distance ourselves from the dregs of judgmentally "wrong behaviors" and treat ourselves to finding out how those differences are "right" for everyone. By choosing to take this broader perspective, we can realign and refocus our sights to discover the potential to be found in a comprehensive, inclusive frame of mind.

This brings us back to the first part of this chapter that lists some of the many phrases and bullet words the media have used to tell us what Asperger's Syndrome is.

Now, we can do away with all the terms that bind AS into a diseased, debilitated, disordered, or ill state. It is not a disease; you cannot catch it and it cannot be cured. "Autism lite" trivializes our subject matter. And let's hold our noses to get past "mental health illness." *Huh?*

Then, let's accept all the phrases and words that suggest difference or alternative way of being. Those that recognize a neurological basis are good. I especially like "neuroexceptional condition."

Next we can slide blithely back to the habitable counsel of Vernon Smith, who gives us a meaningful framework on which to drape our "what is it" of Asperger's Syndrome. Asperger's Syndrome has both deficiencies and advantages, or "selective advantages" that characterize its essence.

Now, with this statement of balance, in nonpejorative terms, we have a clear context in which to explore our AS phenomenon.

Affirmation of Spectrum Core Features

All persons on the autistic spectrum will have difficulty with social interaction, the assigning of emotional/intentional states to self and others in order to understand and predict behavior, and *reciprocal* language. Repetitive or rigid behaviors and absorbing interests. Check, check. These attributes are connate and consistent throughout the autistic spectrum.

Asperger's Syndrome (specifically) Deficiencies and Advantages

Interaction Deficiency. There is not an iota of Asperger's Syndrome information that does not state that the primary deficiency of AS is social interaction. An Aspie simply is not neurologically equipped to be well socialized. His sensory processing tends to note all the details, but misses what those details "mean" to the whole. The social-emotional connection is convoluted, mixed, or unrealized. His emotions/feelings are the same but cannot be expressed, or otherwise worked within a social context. Without a way to read facial expressions and body language, or a way to know what to expect from another's actions, he is left with only literal, straightforward language to try to understand the very complex social world in which other people relate to one another via nonverbal communication.

An Aspie plays with a football on a basketball court. No matter that the Aspie has learned the literal game objective—getting the ball in the basket. No matter if he can calculate how long it will take the ball to get to the basket if it is being shot (oops, that would be "thrown") from a distance of "x" and on a trajectory of "y," it's going to be hard

(I mean, "difficult") to get the double conical football into the round basketball hoop. And the futile attempts are bound to generate anxiety in the Aspie.

He will play his position very well, with precision, having memorized the playbook. But he will play without having absorbed (that would be "understood") the model (that's a "holistic" construct) of team play. He will play without the ability to predict through eye contact, facial expression, and body movement what the other players are doing or are likely to do next, and accordingly, adjust his play options.

Conversely, the neurotypical team, with the basketball, will anticipate and watch every twitch of their teammates' muscles, the timing of every movement of their eyes, and will be able to pass, dribble, turn and feign, react, and adjust their play based on predicting their teammates' corresponding actions. Working together, with a communally understood plan, continuously reading the motion clues as they play, the NTs' strategy of offense and defense will produce, both by plan and by calculated spontaneity, their objective. The Aspie will be fumbling, but he will be thinking and systematizing and . . . (stay tuned)

According to A. Barbour, author of *Louder Than Words: Nonverbal Communication*, "the total impact of a message breaks down like this: 7 percent verbal (words) 38 percent vocal (volume, pitch, rhythm, etc.) and 55 percent body movements (mostly facial expressions)." Both spoken and non spoken language are processed at the same time. Furthermore, it is the *non*verbal language that tells what the verbiage *really* means! Therefore, if one is an Aspie and can hear the words but cannot process the accompanying wordless message found in eye movement, body posture, gestures, touch, personal space, and facial expression as well as in the rhythm, intonation, and stress in the speech, he misses the sum of the *meaning* that the speaker delivers!

When the quality of one's communication is so compromised, as it is for the AS person, what can he do but flounder in frustration on all levels of human contact? What's he to do, avoid everyone? Communicate only by the written word? Relegate himself only "to stand very quietly in a corner, content that he can breathe?" (Franz Kafka)

The quality of interpersonal communication is at the crux of every human-to-human contact. Parent to child, sibling to sibling, student to teacher, passersby, romantic partners. You get the idea. *Together*, we are challenged to unending interface by sharing emotions, learning what is appropriate by cultural standards, understanding everyday social boundaries, and developing our sense of self. Members by birth, we thrive if we know enough about our membership to understand how to make things happen and how to avoid pitfalls. How to cultivate relationships and understand personal boundaries. How to initiate, plan, prioritize, sustain, and predict. How to subconsciously immerse ourselves in our culture's perspective.

It's all a process that we call "socialization." It is what usually just "happens" to us as we grow up in a social unit and participate in the culture's social systems. We are handed a family, a culture, a language, religion, and education. We are able to identify ourselves within the greater social construct. We make friends, advance our well-being through meaningful employment and establish ourselves in an "acceptable" place in the social model. It is expected of us. We get "it," we have "it," we enjoy "it" and we do "it." Indeed, we *are* "it." No one needs to be sat down and taught all the unending details of the values, standards, expectations, limits of behavior, and unwritten rules of one's culture.

No one, that is, who is neurotypical. If, however, one is an Aspie, his brain is not available to take all this in. Instead, he is off enthusiastically learning the facts about his juicy interests, finding his personal bliss in systemizing details or in trying to make sense of the floods of sensory impressions. He does not "get" the gestalt or the big picture of what the NTs are all doing here while maximizing living together, feeling safe and enjoying the aspects of "the team."

The separation of the AS person from being able to "get" all the subtleties of team play constitutes the social deficiency. The AS person is living in the physical social milieu, but is impaired at the interacting, the reciprocation, the manifestation of the *social* self.

Selective Advantages. Though cause and effect have not been determined, Aspie cognition and talent present in an inverse relationship to the quality of social ability. Somewhere, somehow in AS neurology, social challenges trade off with intellectual or artistic gifts. Social deficit + selective advantages = the Aspie paradox.

It is inherent to the AS identity that Aspies will have normal to genius levels of intelligence, and often, remarkable talent in art, music, literature, math, physics, or articulation of ideals. Remember, there is no cognitive delay in AS. Matter of fact, Aspies are the ones we most often credit with our scientific, technical, and cultural evolution.

News.bbc.co.uk reporter Megan Lane asks, "What is the link between this condition and creativity, be it in the arts or sciences?" Professor Michael Fitzgerald of Dublin's Trinity College: "People with it are generally hyper focused, very persistent workaholics who tend to see things from detail to global rather than looking at the bigger picture first and then working backwards, as most people do." And, according to Ms. Lane, Professor Simon Baron-Cohen of Cambridge University says "it is more accurate to describe this creativity as 'systemising'—a strong drive to analyze detail. This might be in mathematics, machines, natural phenomena or anatomy, to identify rules that govern a system and any variations in that system."[3]

Professor Fitzgerald also states that "many leading figures in the fields of science, politics and the arts have achieved success because they had autistic spectrum disorder," believing that there is a relationship between autism and genius.

Several sources quote Hans Asperger as believing that "for success in science or art, a dash of autism is essential. The essential ingredient may be an ability to turn away from the everyday world, from the simply practical and to rethink a subject with originality so as to create in new untrodden ways with all abilities canalized into the one specialty."

(Back to our football/basketball game) . . . *may become fascinated with some detail of the basket, the angles, points and texture of the ball, the ball's arc of trajectory or the crossed lines of the net, or the interface of shadows cast by the pole, net and rim and the wood of the floor. The Aspie with the football in the basketball arena may, with focused genius on some narrow intense interest, rethink all the obvious data and come up with some as yet unfathomed solution, perspective or invention that will cause all the other players to marvel, and will perhaps advance the game to a whole new dimension.*

Additional Assets

Because the AS person lacks internalized social ability, he, correspondingly, is not apt to assimilate the myriad social games that NTs play. Often, that's a good thing. In the AS person's case, it allows him to possess many ideals of behavior that can be reconciled, appreciated, and valued by the majority of neurotypical persons.

To wit: Being that an Aspie neither detects in others nor knows how to play social games, even for self-preservation, he will be **truthful**. Ask a question, he will give you an honest answer, even if it is not to his (socialized) advantage to do so. Blame him for something and he won't get defensive. If he did it, he will say so.

Among other "games" he likely does *not* play is exploitation—taking advantage of others' weaknesses. He has **no interest in hurting others** or in being a bully. Manipulation of others is an alien concept; he is not inclined to attack the reputation of those around him. He does not pressure anyone. He has **no hidden agendas**, no social subterfuge. He is who he says he is and does what he says he will do.

He is **nonjudgmental**, free of prejudice for age, race, gender or other cosmetic criteria, and will typically enjoy the idiosyncrasies of others.

Add to this integrity; he is **honest, loyal, trustworthy, sincere, and dependable**.

He is not demanding **(not a whiner!)** and can **entertain himself** for hours.

He is **psychologically independent**; not likely to be influenced by social convention or financial or political pressures.

He **loves knowledge**, is curious, and will pursue his interests with **focus, fervor,** and **perseverance. Accountability**, check.

Can we be more clear that the Aspie is a **reliable friend** if you don't want or need reciprocity too far outside of a shared interest? A **stable and faithful partner** if you are a nurturer or a giver and are not emotionally needy yourself? A **smart, dependable employee** if you don't need one with a socially interactive agenda?

Hidden Probabilities

As with the proverbial iceberg, the observable behaviors of an AS person are worthy of discovery, but Aspies, like NTs, are very complex. In addition to the socially observable features of AS, we recognize several other neurological operatives.

The Aspie personality ensemble would likely include **sensory integration and processing issues**. Hyper or hyposensitivity to light, sound, taste, smell, texture, touch, and pain are common. He might have difficulty hearing auditory detail or sorting out which sound, when there are several at once, is the relevant sound to listen to. It may take extra time for him to figure out which meaning, of a word with several meanings, is intended. For example, he might be miffed hearing the word "charged." Is the meaning like, being "charged" with an offense, or like a battery being "charged," or like a credit card being "charged," or like an opponent being "charged" or the air being "charged" with electricity?

He might be **restless, intense,** and have a long attention span in the area of his interests.

Feeling **social anxiety** is typical; panic attacks and phobias may be present.

He might well question the status quo and **resist direction**. Flatly put, he doesn't like to be told what to do.

He probably has a strong need to **organize the experience of his world**, both in his physical environment and in his daily routines. He will become **anxious** if unanticipated change has to be made.

Fixed ideas may determine behavior. Rigid adherence to a personal standard or idea may control a behavior despite outside rationale to the contrary.

Aspies are exacting and love **correcting** misstatement or error. "The blue-eyed white alligator is not albino, it is leucistic." The need is for accuracy both for themselves and for others.

He is **vulnerable** to anyone attempting to "use" him for their own gain.

In his **naiveté** he will **seem younger than he** is, almost childlike.

He will **score very well on IQ tests**. Ability to systemize and identify sequencing and patterns are scoreable talents on these cognitive ability tests.

He likely will have a difficult time expressing his emotion or understanding the emotional and communication signals of others. He cannot gauge another's interest as they speak. He may have impaired comprehension, including **misinterpretation** of another's meaning. He may say, *"Wait, what do you mean?"*

Sensing that his social experience is somehow at odds with others, he may feel **isolated**.

He will **lack "executive" skills**. These include initiating, projecting, planning, prioritizing, strategizing, monitoring. He lacks intention and behavioral control. He likely cannot direct his behavior to accomplish goals or objectives.

He will **not have expectations** of others. If an AS person is financially successful in terms of employment or independent achievement, it is usually because it passively "happens" to him, or he is "discovered" rather than by proactive pursuit of financial or career development.

Memory of details, locations, or facts is one valuable Aspie facet.

He has a **unique perspective in nonsocial problem solving**.

Perhaps the most difficult and subtle operational feature of Aspie behavior is that he likely has not socialized the **appropriate boundaries** for behavior. It is the lack of knowledge about unspoken boundaries and lack of recognition of social models for given situations that plague those in Aspiedom. NTs will likely notice the AS lack of conformity and identify him as goofy or retarded not to know better.

It is a boundaries issue when a young adult Aspie is encouraged by acquaintances in a bar to go talk to a woman he finds attractive. As small talk is difficult, the Aspie just grabs her instead! It is a boundaries issue when an adult Aspie male tackles his married adult sister as though they were rough housing eight-year-olds. It is a boundaries issue when the married Aspie does not recognize the threat posed to his marriage by his wife's continued interest in and sharing of time with a male coworker. It is a boundaries issue when a single male Aspie repeatedly compliments ("hits" on) his married coworker despite her repeated mention to him of her husband. It was a boundaries issue when preteen Aspie Dylan drew Easter bunnies with their heads being exploded off their bodies, or wrote and graphically illustrated a book of violent poems, or as an adult said to a gift-giver, "Next time just give me the money instead!"

Having an unorthodox or otherwise **special interest** is a paramount feature of those in Aspiedom. The fascination or even "obsession" is usually asocial, restricted, pertains to a body of knowledge about the favored subject, and will exclude interest in other subjects. It is often age inappropriate, such as a second grader engrossed with one of the World Wars, or topically oblique, such as an interest in nostrils. The interest may be short term or it may last a lifetime. One may adopt a few interests at a time or they may be serially changeable. The interest may grow into a career, an invention or to scientific discovery.

This special interest is, no doubt, one of the selective advantages of Aspiedom. And it may be the self-cure for social angst. When one's attention is absorbed by an enthralling interest, one does not have to make any annoying social considerations; the confusion of constantly trying to read or figure out what is going on socially will disappear, and the Aspie will be free to explore a delicious treat of flight all on his own, finding freedom and calmness in his otherwise anxious existence. Think of the incredible release in being able to dissolve into and completely indulge in something one loves! And yes, he may find something there that no one else has seen before.

Coexisting Phenomena

Clinging to and hanging about the nuclear aspects of Aspiedom are a host of coexisting phenomena. We see complications and complexities. According to Stephen Bauer, MS MPH, Asperger's Syndrome often presents with other types of diagnoses, including: "tic disorders such as **Tourette disorder, attentional problems** and mood problems such as **depression** and **anxiety**."[4] And according to G. Robert DeLong and Judith T. Dwyer, Duke University Medical Center, the rate of bipolar affective disorder "is significantly higher in families with Asperger's Syndrome."[5] Also, very commonly concurring is **O**bsessive-**C**ompulsive **D**isorder. Other concomitant conditions include **O**ppositional **D**efiant **D**isorder, **A**nxiety **D**isorder, **B**orderline **P**ersonality **D**isorder, **S**leep **D**isorder, and **A**ggression. They may have **dyspraxia** (clumsiness), **dysphasia** (difficulty speaking), **dyslexia** (difficulty interpreting letters or words), **hyperlexia** (extreme reading, advanced vocabulary, interest in words), **prosophagnosia** (face blindness), or **synasthesia** (thinking in pictures, textures, shapes or colors, or in strings of information).

Often, more than one of these conditions will attend the Aspie. They may be secondary to the neurological condition or an integral part thereof. Some are problematic, some are not. It is these features that render each Asperger's Syndrome person different than another. These and the multistrength nature of the spectrum itself.

Disability?

"Physical Disability." "Mental Disability." We're familiar with these concepts and accept their inclusion into the social tapestry, but "Interactive Disability?" We are not conceptually there yet. For children being diagnosed as Asperger's Syndrome persons, the need for educational and social accommodations *is* being realized. But for adults identifying with AS, much is yet to be done. For the most part, until social awareness is increased, the adult Aspie is left in varying degrees to accommodate on his own.

Life is difficult for the Aspie, especially if he has no way of knowing everything that he, by NT standards, needs to know to be a productive adult. Indeed, he might not even know what "socially productive" means or that being productive is socially valued. And it is yet more difficult if he realizes that somehow he is different, or perhaps something is "wrong" *but doesn't know what is wrong* or *in what way* he is different.

In talking about the Asperger's identity in our neurotypical midst, we have to be mindful that the concept of disability is very difficult for a culture to grasp when there is *no physical indication* of that disability. There are no wheelchairs, canes, crutches, or seeing-eye dogs. There are no missing limbs or bodily disfigurement.

And not to be forgotten, an Aspie score on an IQ test would no doubt put him *well above* the score of 70, below which is an accepted standard for intellectual disability. Conversely, an Aspie's score would likely place him in the range of scores where no one could understand why, for goodness' sake, someone so smart would claim any impairment of any kind! "Interactive Disability" is a concept that will not be readily accepted into the prevailing lexicon.

But an average or high IQ does not tell the whole story and *does not negate disability*. Nor is there any formal definition or other current measurement for interactive disability or impairment. Aspies are left completely out of the loop when it comes to traditional social standards of disability. Thus, Asperger's Syndrome is sometimes referred to as the "invisible autism," and by extension, the invisible disability.

From having serious qualitative social issues and at the same time, often, gifts, AS does in fact present differently from person to person. In some cases, there is disablement, in some cases there are gifts, and most likely, both are present.

No doubt about social impairment. Whether that amounts to a disability is a matter of how well one functions. A top-tier Aspie could be completely independent. He could be living as an adult in an NT social construct. He, having found suitable employment, a life partner, perhaps a family, would not by any contemporary standards be considered disabled.

Another AS person may live independently, but not be functioning with adult credentials. He may suffer in a world where people use vague and subtle communication like facial expressions and body language he cannot "read." He may find some work but likely will be underemployed in terms of his education, talent, or interests. He probably has repeated failures in aligning a romantic partner. He may have children but will not be able to make the expected bond with them or perform the leadership role of a parent. He may have some dysfunction in the adult areas of planning finances, securing bank accounts, filing tax returns, and being insured. In this scenario, there is a significant degree of social dysfunction. With appropriate support, this person no doubt could find fulfilling employment and get up to speed with forms and paperwork necessary to establish an adult identity. No doubt about social deficits here, but should we call the lacks or misses a disability?

On yet another level, an Aspie, in the face of repeated social failures, may retreat into isolation, becoming derelict. Disability?

And there are others who, if they had identified with Asperger's Syndrome and had appropriate social support, might not have given up and disappeared into the abyss of suicide. Were these persons disabled?

So the tough social questions revolve around how to identify the need and how to provide corresponding support. Even if we accept "Interactive Disability" as a viable concern, we are faced with what to do with it. How do we measure it? What kind of accommodations are needed? Who will pay for it? What can we expect it to accomplish? What will such a tag mean to the bearer? Can one be both disabled and enabled?

Colloquial as it is, disability is as disability does. At present, we have no clear, consistent guidelines for assessing or addressing either the scope of impairment or the degree thereof. The Aspie is challenged to function the best he can, despite society's lack of recognition that AS persons do not operate with neurotypical brains and do not socialize the same as do NTs.

Compounding the issue is the fact that most social agencies that might be of help to an AS person require that one needing assistance must be proactive, "own" their situation, and *ask for help*. This process of asking another person or agency for help is a construct of socialization that neurotypicals take for granted. But for an AS person, who has not developed that social model, how would he know what to do, what to say, where to go, what to expect by asking for help? Given what we know about our Asperger's person, there is no chance that on his own he would even have a clue as to what "help" could mean to him. Is the *inability* to ask for help a *disability*?

Ultimately, despite the continuing throwing about of brains, as contemporary culture increasingly recognizes Aspiedom, we may begin to reduce problematic behaviors and increase the social benefits afforded by these exceptional persons. Unorthodox social functioning may yet be celebrated . . . .

WHAT DOES IT LOOK LIKE?

"What a piece of work is man!"

—Hamlet

Observable Aspie Essence

The sets of behavioral and physical markers that consistently occur together easily tell the Asperger's Syndrome tale. Once learned, a casual but aware observer can discover and appreciate Aspies everywhere.

The experience is like reading the children's book *Where's Waldo?* by Martin Hanford. The reader goes on an adventure, trying to find Waldo, who is obscured by very detailed drawings of large crowds of people. It is only because one knows that Waldo wears a red and white striped long-sleeved pullover shirt, a red and white pom-pom hat and glasses that he can be discerned from the rest of the crowd. But the reader must study the picture carefully before he can self-reward with, "There he is!"

Finding an Aspie is all about knowing the raiment of one in Aspiedom—knowing what to look for. Horizontally, they are in crowds we see every day. Vertically, they are among everyone we have ever seen, known or experienced; they are banked in our memory. We have AS persons around us on a day-to-day basis and we have AS persons in our past experience. We can identify both by observing today and by remembering yesterday.

The most salient aspect of an Aspie is that he appears *at once* "odd" and remarkably "smart." So if you know or remember someone like that, you have a good start on recognizing an AS person. We, too, sense a social awkwardness in him, but probably cannot put a finger on our discernment until we take a closer look. So for further consideration, we scrutinize the individual physical traits as well as the interactive behavior to identify an AS person.

Gait trait. The way an AS person walks may be distinguishing, such as on the balls of the feet instead of having the heel touch first with each step. In the literature, the exaggerated term for these persons is "toe walkers." Other gait features may be a slight jarring at the end of each step, a sense of body hardness, rigidity, or bobbing up and down. The gait may be asymmetrical, with one arm swinging more than the other, or both arms may simply be left hanging at one's side instead of moving alternately with the legs. Hands may be kept in pockets or held together behind the back as one walks. The Aspie often walks looking down, immediately in front of him.

Dystonia. Unusual muscle tone noted particularly in the exptremities. Hypo- or hypertonia may account for postural and gait anomalies and rigidity or limpness of limbs. It may play a role in the "clumsiness" often noted in AS persons.

Use of eyes. Eye contact will be avoided while walking toward others, such as through a hall, even at a workplace when all the potential encounters are familiar people. He won't initiate "Hi" as he sees you in the hall or on the street. When he is conversing with someone he will most often avoid the other person's eyes, especially when he is talking. He may quickly and occasionally glance at the other person, or look at them out of the corner of his eyes. His eyes may dart off for no apparent reason, or stare, or he may look at the speaker's mouth instead of his eyes. While neurotypical persons characteristically use a mix of holding and furtive glances to communicate, the Aspie does not demonstrate knowledge of these subtle conversational cues. Several YouTube videos featuring Aspies demonstrate this feature.

Use of fingers. I've noticed, viewing AS persons in real life and on YouTube, that they often will use their fingers atypically. One videotaped person explains a detail of her artwork using all five fingers spread widely apart instead of using the expected pointing of a single finger. On another video, the camera shows a person's fingers of both hands being repeatedly loosely woven together then taken apart, in sync with his rhythm of speech. The finger movements are meaningless in terms of adding expression to the verbalization.

Repetitive movement. Most Aspies will have a signature repetition of movement, thought to reduce anxiety. However, over time, an adult generally will have learned not to "stim" in public so as not to draw attention to himself. The most common of these repetitive movements is rocking. I have seen this in the workplace where ergonomic chairs have a tilt-back option that allows for a rocking movement. I also recently saw someone I identified as an AS person repetitively squeezing with one hand the first and fourth fingers across the top of the middle two fingers of his other hand. Right hand squeezed the left fingers, then left hand squeezed the right. And again, and again.

Speaking anomalies. The Aspie will have a difficult time with small talk. He may butt into or blurt out into conversation or may dominate it with a "download" of information that may or may not be related to the topic at hand. He may not know when it is his turn to speak. Or he may just blurt out a one-liner.

Verbal ability. Often, an AS person will have very developed verbal skills, especially if he is talking about his area of expertise or interest, but he will have difficulty in the expression of language as used in reciprocal conversation. I had to marvel the first time I heard, in my workplace, a nearly mute and very socially remote person speak, in this case to a supervisor, about a work detail. I could tell by her precise, formal vocabulary and perfect English that she was very intelligent. Based on the observed elements of social muteness, complete avoidance of eye contact, intelligence, and formal speech (as needed and still without eye contact), I concluded that she is an AS person.

Facial expression. Facial expression may be cheerless, flat, or held too long, such as a smile that gets pasted on, or doesn't relax soon enough. AS persons may appear puzzled with what someone else is saying, particularly if the speaker is unexpectedly using figurative speech or is not presenting linear dialog where one complete sentence logically follows another. Or if the speaker changes subjects too quickly.

Solitary. No water-cooler conversationalist here. Our AS adult will take breaks from work and eat lunch, even in a cafeteria setting, by himself, probably reading. Unless, of course, he is trying to connect socially, not having given up on relationships. He may sit beside or just sort of hang on to familiar people without contributing depth or movement to a conversation. The people who are convenient to sit by at the lunch table will probably not be hanging out together off the work site, however. The Aspie will usually be considered a loner; he does not have a circle of friends.

Lack of social convention. He will show little regard for contemporary ideas of style, and will not dress or groom himself to please anyone else. His clothing will be a uniform that is a product of comfort for the individual. His hair style may remain constant for years.

Will seem aloof, egocentric to others. The Aspie just doesn't have a clue as to how to initiate conversation or forge friendships, even though he may desperately want to. Despite appearances, he is not "stuck up."

Behavior that demonstrates lack of social boundaries. He may react to any situation in an atypical way, thereby surprising the neurotypical person who has learned what is and what is not acceptable behavior.

Routines, repetitive behavior patterns. One Aspie I've observed eats the same thing in the work cafeteria daily. He opens a paper napkin, places it horizontally on the table, then lines up his three hard-boiled eggs on it and eats them one by one from left to right!

Tics. Sometimes part of the "odd" essence of an Aspie is a muscle or vocal tic. This can result in a facial grimace or too rapid blinking or squeezing shut of the eyes; it may present as a grunt or clearing of the throat.

Unusual voice prosody. An Aspie's speech may be choppy, mistimed, monotonic, or flat. His volume might be a little loud, as though he were hard of hearing. As voice rhythms, volume, and intonation are learned through "reading" the expression of others, an Aspie may miss the expressive elements of speech and thereby speak peculiarly.

If the Asperger person has found suitable employment, it will be where his talents with computers or other technology can be utilized, where he can perform expected and clearly delineated tasks, and where very little social interaction is required. He will excel in fields where being a "people person" is not important, such as programming, architecture, accounting, and engineering.

My personal discovery of other adult AS persons came from the Aspie-friendly environment where I recently worked. No ability at job interviewing was needed. The employment requirement was simply that one have at least a bachelor's degree from an accredited college. (Subsequently, though, on-the-job performance criteria had to be met.) Each of the four hundred persons sat at a computer in his own cubicle and electronically scored written or interpretive responses to standardized testing for school children. He used his "smarts" to score communication arts, math, and science. And he usually scored accurately, thereby justifying his hire. His attention to detail and his dependability were appreciated. He could work without talking to anyone and without anyone else bothering him. He didn't have to "kiss up" to anyone, and it didn't matter if he stared, rocked, walked with a funny gait, dressed in a "uniform" of comfort, or didn't socialize at all. Scoring was done for 7.25 hours a day, on a seasonal basis. Breaks and lunch were on schedule. Everyone knew what to expect and routinely performed the tasks. Only occasionally would one need to interact with a supervisor.

Another place where one may find an AS person would be at the gym or track. Any activity that requires endurance, individual focus, and concentration will attract an adult Aspie.

And as Aspies are frequently avid readers who enjoy the acquisition of information, they may be found studying a favorite subject in a library or on a computer, or they may be enrapt in their favorite fiction.

Casual observation of someone walking down the street probably will not affirm a presence in Aspiedom. However, one may get a positive read in only a brief encounter by observing repeated motion, awkward interaction and unusual eye movement of a possible AS person.

Not long ago, I had the opportunity to visit a large aquarium where guides were positioned at various stations to tell visitors about their subject on display. In this case, our family of four was viewing a white alligator. The guide was the person mentioned earlier who was alternately squeezing the fingers on one hand then the other. He did not offer information until I asked about the "albino" reptile. He looked at me briefly, but his eyes quickly averted as he set into his spiel that the alligator was not "albino." He pointed out that it did not have pink eyes, that in fact it had blue eyes, some pale pigment and instead was "leucistic."

Though the narrator's interactive skills were not great, he was functioning and no doubt enjoying his subject, if not the personal interaction. Dylan and I agreed that here was another Aspie. The repetitive motion or "stimming" of squeezing the fingers together, the lack of conversational initiative, his averted eyes, the minilecture correction of my "albino" misstatement, all within a scientific context, added up to our discovery. The other two persons in the party, Dylan's daughter, Brittney, and Mike, were a little reserved about our bold "Aspie" claim after a barely two-minute meeting.

And we can't leave this chapter without noting, too, that the identification of an AS person may not come by contemplating the "piece of work" that is someone else. The identification may come through the solo act of reading—reading about the behaviors, traits, and attributes of one in Aspiedom, then finding a definitive personal fit . . . .

UNFOLDED ASPIES

"To be or not to be, that is the question."
—Hamlet

After realizing that Dylan resided in Aspiedom, I began to discover AS persons everywhere. I found them in my workplace (the count is eight, out of about four hundred), then I found one in my ninety-year-old uncle, in one of my cousins, and in the plumber. One lives down the block.

After my explanation about what Asperger's Syndrome is, a friend realized that her son-in-law must have Asperger's Syndrome. Likewise, my chiropractor recognized his cousin as an Aspie. My handyman contractor said that everything I mentioned about Asperger's Syndrome fits his friend, who has unusual interests in jet skis; you know, like getting excited about knowing all the data available on the Internet of exactly the size and number of holes in the jets from 1968 to today.

The list goes on—our waitress's brother, a dinner guest's brother, a friend of a friend. Almost everyone I talk to about AS knows someone who fits my descriptions. And you will too.

And I have finally, from a memory more than fifty years old, identified as an AS person the quiet oaf from my childhood Sunday school class who, for no apparent reason, pinched me *really* hard. I remember two

Aspies from my public-school years. From my young adult years, I now identify, as an AS person, a medical student I dated.

My contention is that with even a marginally "trained eye" and in any social situation, without knowing history or taking an interview, you and I can, with considerable assuredness, discern an AS person. By the time you finish this book, you will no doubt be seeing Aspies around you. And if you have so isolated yourself that there is no one around you, the AS person probably is *you*.

Meet Them: Aspies from Memory

LL is the Sunday-school idiot nerd thug with the nasty pinching fingers, whose bad behavior was dismissed by the adult teachers who told me that the offense was **LL**'s way of showing me that he liked me! What? Well, I can, with my new AS awareness, finally forgive both the Sunday school pinch and the pedagogic brush off. I hope **LL** and the teachers can forgive me for my previous disagreeable thoughts thereof.

SW: In elementary school, **SW** was rumored to have stabbed a pet with a knife; he seemed sullen and aloof, and most kids steered clear of him. By eighth grade, I'm embarrassed (now) to say that some of we "cooler" students elected scary, mostly silent **SW** to eighth-grade Science class president as a joke so we could laugh at his new "popularity" and be entertained by watching him grope for words to begin or dismiss the class session.

JS: In Junior High, **JS** was academic, but also "out of it," as demonstrated by her coarse laugh, which left her mouth open and her eyes staring long after such a response was appropriate. Smart as she was, nobody but a real weirdo would have a grunting laugh like that, then just leave their mouth agape and stare, wondering what to do next. And her mother, always hanging around, was equally dense. Now that I think about it, Mom was probably an Aspie too! Boy, did the two of them seem out of it to the more popular and struggling to be popular (myself) girls . . . .

SH: Medical school was the obvious choice for someone so fascinated by "tissue" (I don't mean paper). As a girlfriend, I was impressed that **SH** seemed so dedicated to his particular interest, and I did enjoy touring the medical school on our cadaver date, seeing those dissected dead people and the fetuses in formaldehyde. Some very interesting tissue there! He and I never really connected emotionally, but I always respected him and was struck by his "brights" and a certain profundity about him. His twinkie gait (slight toe-walking) did not plus me at all, so I just kind of ignored it; that, and his grimace-like smile were at least doable.

I am humbled by my new knowledge of Asperger's Syndrome and hope that **LL, SW, JS,** and **SH** have found satisfying lives for themselves. If they haven't yet been (other- or self-) identified as AS persons I hope that they can, as soon as possible, realize that they are validated in Aspiedom. I ask that they accept my apologies for my insensitivity from many years ago.

Meet Them: Current

JP: The plumber. He is the only one who can really figure out the best way to facilitate repairs in a century-old home, with its antique plumbing concepts and fixtures. And he does stare, but only for the few seconds he dares to make eye contact. Yes, he is odd, with speech that is too loud and with pauses in the wrong places. At first, I thought he must be deaf, but now I get the whole picture, including why he would rather have me go to the plumbing stores to get the parts he specifies, instead of doing it himself—he does not want to try to communicate with the clerks. A missed communication was no doubt the basis of a "run in" he told me about with one plumbing supplier. Another supplier commented to me that **JP** didn't seem like the "sharpest tack in the box." Au contraire! What I know now is that those suppliers just have no idea of who he is, and would rather put him down so that they look like the smarties. Whoa! It's **JP**, with his sharpness, I'll call on when we need to solve the next plumbing problem.

BS lives down the block. He seems lonely and begins talking "at" any recognizable person from the neighborhood who is out and about. Unless I have time to spare, I've learned to avoid him, as I haven't figured out how to let him know when the conversation is over, when I need to move along. He only talks about himself, just stringing it all out, not stopping even when I try to excuse myself with, "Talk to you later," then, "It was nice to see you," and finally, "I *have* to go." There is no reciprocal conversation, it's totally **BS**'s download—on and on and on. I struggle to pull myself away and still be polite, but he just keeps talking! I nod to concur with whatever he is saying as I start on my way, opting out of trying to dismiss myself again. If I hadn't recently recognized him as Aspie, I'd definitely think that he was passive aggressive, and I would feel affronted that he should be so free as to put me in the position of being the baddie by walking away from him.

Eight persons at my recent workplace: One appears to be anorexic. Two are female. Three races are represented. Two are quite tall, no one is overweight. Hair color ranges from red to brown to black, from kinky to straight. Facial expressions are mostly "flat"; one stares, two always look down, effectively avoiding eye contact with anyone. Only one hangs around at a regular time with one or two other people. The jarring and ball-of-foot walking styles are represented. From comments I overheard, I recognize one person to be very emotionally depressed. The ages range from about thirty-five to sixty; I say this with the caveat that I am not particularly good at guessing age and that Aspies often appear younger than their year of birth might indicate. There isn't a neurotypical working there who, like me, would not see any of these eight persons as "odd" or "eccentric."

I have the ultimate respect for these AS persons I recognize in my daily life and in the workplace. I do not want to offend them in any way. I continue to pursue making Asperger's information available to everyone with whom I come in contact and recognize as an AS person. My calling is to help them find a satisfying identity for themselves and relieve them of their (usually) known social disparateness by providing them with materials that give an explanation that will make sense to their logical minds.

Of the five Aspies at work I have approached with Asperger's Syndrome information, not one had heard of it. One was not interested in hearing about it. Two others thanked me for giving them information. One has given me a response to verify that the information about "socialization" does describe him. As to the other three, I'm still looking for the right opportunity to approach them with, "Have you ever heard of Asperger's Syndrome?" Ditto for **JP** the Plumber and **BS** the Talker—if I can get a word in edgewise . . . .

CAUSES/EFFECTS/ WHAT'S GOING ON

"Being nature's livery, or fortune's star . . ."
—Hamlet

Everyone wants to know what causes Asperger's Syndrome, especially parents, including parents with *grown* children. With good reason too. Because of *their own* social programming, parents are bewildered, worried, and feel guilty about being responsible for their child's emotional difficulties, behavior, failure to conform, or failure to succeed in the ways they or others expect of them.

From coursework as a psychology major in college and through my continued less formal study in behavior, human potential, and child rearing, I submit that the prevailing theory to date has been that parents are the ones responsible for how their children behave and how they "turn out." According to this functional theory, it is Mom and Dad who are answerable when problematic or atypical behaviors are exhibited by their offspring. They are charged with failing to socialize their children properly.

While recognizing that not all parenting is of equal quality and *is* particularly influential in rearing neurotypical children, I now also realize that a person's neurology may be the genesis for behavior. The traditional standards that judge parenting may not apply. This alternative consideration is especially indicated when one child's behavior is very incongruous with the behavior of his siblings and disparate from family history and the role modeling provided by the parents. One child follows and thrives in the familial social model and another does not.

With awareness of Asperger's Syndrome, we now know that many behaviors *are* brain based. Parents of AS persons can set aside the myopic functional paradigm that automatically charges them with emotional deprivation, abuse or otherwise poor parenting and instead look to neural function to account for unique behaviors.

Once we accept the theory that an alternative neurology manifests in alternative behavior, we become hungry to know more about what makes the AS person's brain different from the neurotypical brain. Both research and cogitation go on and on to uncover anomalies of cause. Hypotheses range from prenatal influences and birth trauma to postnatal environmental insult, genetic throwbacks, and alien intervention. Answers do not come easily . . . .

Prenatal Environment

- *Extreme Male Brain:* Dr. Bonnie Auyeung, Professor Simon Baron-Cohen and colleagues at Cambridge University have found an association between fetal testosterone and autistic traits, indicating that higher testosterone levels in the womb "not only masculinizes the body, it masculinizes the mind and therefore the brain." This leads to male neurological qualities such as a "much stronger drive towards analysis and constructing systems and can have a great ability to focus on something that absorbs them."[1]

- *Maternal levels of glutathione and homocysteine:* A recent study by Dr. Jill James of the Autism Speaks' Autism Treatment Network shows that "low levels of glutathione, coupled with high production levels of another chemical, homocysteine, greatly increase the chances of a woman having a child with Autism."[2]

- *Genes that govern "natural killer" immune cells:* Dr. Jeffrey Gregg and researchers at University of California, Davis, found eleven of these genes that are more active in autistic children. The detection bolsters theories that "some sort of infectious agent, early in life or even in the womb might play a role in autism."[3]

- *Cytokines: It is known that cytokines affect mood and behavior.* "In autistic children neuroglial cells produce cytokines in an unbalanced fashion. This can lead to inflammatory changes in the brain, which in turn can affect development and behavior," according to scientists at Johns Hopkins University.[4]

Congenital Influence

- *Birth Trauma:* According to Dr. Viola Frymann, an osteopathic physician, birth trauma is the most common cause of developmental problems, including autism, attention deficits, and learning disabilities. "Problems in delivery resulting from the skull compression of birthing can affect the brain and spinal column as well as the fluids that are inside. The insult is thus on the nervous system . . ."[5]

Physical/Circumstantial Environment

- *Paternal age:* A team of American and British experts, led by Dr. Abraham Reichenberg, publishing in the September 2006 edition of the *Archives of General Psychiatry*, said that "children born to men older than 40 had a six times higher risk of being autistic than those born to men under 30. The researchers suggest there may be a genetic fault which is more common with age. "This might be spontaneous mutations in sperm-producing cells or alterations in genetic 'imprinting,' which affects gene expression."[6]

- *Maternal age*: University of California researchers say that "a 40-year-old woman's risk of having a child later diagnosed with autism is 50 percent greater than that of a woman between 25 and 29 years old." They also found that advanced paternal age is associated with higher autism risk only when the father is older and the mother is under 30.[7]

- *Rainfall rates:* Michael Waldman of Cornell University recently published a study that correlates an increase in rainfall to an increase in autism diagnoses. The study involved children born between 1987 and 1999 in California, Oregon, and Washington (diagnosed in 2005) and rainfall rates from 1987 to 2001.[8]

- *Aborted baby DNA:* A study by the Environmental Protection Agency indicates that the year autism rates increased dramatically coincides with the year that "a second dose of the MMR vaccine, which included cells derived from aborted baby tissue, was being recommended." The aborted fetal tissue introduced to youngsters by vaccine may be involved in an autoimmune response that "may be involved in the etiology of autism."[9]

- *Toxic Exposure:* Many sources point to heavy metal contamination during infancy. Mercury, lead, and ethanol are established as neurotoxins that lead to developmental issues. Childhood vaccinations, especially those containing the preservative Thimerosal, have been widely accused of causing autism. In the USA, vaccines are no longer made with this additive.

Recent Brain Research Projects

- *Structural:* The Society for Neuroscience reviewed a study that showed "individuals with Asperger's Syndrome had bilateral shape abnormalities in the intraparietal sulcus that correlated with age, intelligence quotient, and . . . social and repetitive behavior scores . . . ." The findings were consistent with evidence of an altered trajectory of early brain development in autism."[10]

Researchers from the University of California, Davis, found that autistic males (females were not included in this study) "suffer from a diminished number of neurons in their amygdala. They found that although there was no variance among amygdala volumes in all the brains, the autistic males as a group had roughly 1.5 million fewer neurons than their peers."[11]

One study using sophisticated imaging techniques led by Manzar Ashtari of the Children's Hospital of Philadelphia found that "autistic children have enlarged gray matter in parietal lobes of the brain linked to the *mirror neuron system* of cells associated with empathy, emotional experience and learning through sight.

"Those children also showed a decrease in gray matter volume in the right amygdala region of the brain that correlated with degrees of impairment in social interaction."[12]

- *Lack of connectivity among certain areas of the brain:* "Using functional magnetic resonance imaging, a team of researchers affiliated with the University of Washington's Autism Center found that the "most severely socially impaired subjects in the study . . . exhibited the most abnormal pattern of connectivity among a network of brain regions involved in face processing."[13]

And from City University, London, UK, "We suggest that ASD may be characterized by atypicalities in the integration of physiological and cognitive aspects of emotional experiences which we argue arise because of poor connectivity between the amygdala and functionally associated cortical areas."[14]

Two proteins, neurologin-1 and neurologin-2, create physical bridges at the synapses of nerve cells that enable them to make connections, or "talk to" other nerve cells. One theory, based on a study at the University of Texas, asserts that autism involves an "imbalance between excitatory and inhibitory connections."[15]

In various other studies, the amounts of dopamine, epinephrine, serotonin, and oxytocin have been implicated in neural connectivity.

- *Slower auditory processing:* "Children with autism spectrum disorders process sound and language a fraction of a second slower than children without ASDs," found a study at Children's Hospital of Philadelphia. "The auditory system may be slower to develop and mature. It means that a child with ASD, on hearing the word 'elephant,' is still processing the 'el' sound while other children have moved on. The delays cascade as a conversation progresses, and the child may lag behind typically developing peers." This is an important finding because if that delay can be accurately measured using magnetic signals, it could become a way to scientifically diagnose autism.[16]

Genetics

- *Clock genes:* Scientists in Wales, led by Dr. Dawn Wimpory, reported that autism is associated with two genes involved in timing and biological clocks. These genes control "sleep cycle, memory and communicative timing." The hypothesis is that a deficiency in social timing contributes to the difficulties faced by people with autism.[17]

- *Lingering Lyonization:* Christopher Robert Badcock, PhD, reports that accidentally retained X chromosome inactivation could explain Asperger's Syndrome. "X-inactivation imprints placed on specific X genes in a woman's body might be accidentally retained on the X chromosome she passed on to her children."[18]

- *Solely genetic:* Michael Wigler at Cold Spring Harbor Laboratory in New York considers autism "entirely genetic." He emphasizes that genetics are hugely complex, involving as many as two hundred genes, and that how they translate into behaviors is not yet understood.[19]

- *Gene identity:* Researchers from the Autism Research Center in Cambridge have linked to Asperger's Syndrome twenty-seven genes that "represent preliminary leads for understanding the genetic bases of AS and related traits, such as empathy . . . ."[20]

In 2004, Finnish researchers associated AS with nine stretches of DNA on six different chromosomes.[21]

Researchers from Johns Hopkins University pinpointed a rogue gene—CNTNAP2—that raises the risk of autism. It is one of more than thirty genes that have been linked to the condition. "This gene makes a protein that helps brain cells communicate with each other and is also thought to be involved in brain development."[22]

- *Genetic variant:* "Researchers have identified a gene variant that is associated with both autism and gastrointestinal problems in individuals with autism." Because this MET C gene is involved with both brain development and how the gastrointestinal system works, and because 30 to 70 percent of children with autism have gastro-intestinal problems, they think they may have identified one factor in an autism sub-type.[23]

- *Mutation:* Dr. Norio Ozaki and colleagues of Fujita Health University School of Medicine in Japan have found a mutation of the gene called the human serotonin transporter gene, hSERT. The gene helps control how the body uses serotonin, a message-carrying chemical or neurotransmitter linked with mood. "Six of the seven people with the mutation had an obsessive-compulsive disorder; some also had anorexia, Asperger's Syndrome . . . social phobia, or were abusers of alcohol."[24]

- *Chromosomal duplication or deletion:* The Autism Consortium in Boston found that "children with a duplicated or missing segment of chromosome 16, which appears to control certain brain functions, have a risk for autism 100 times greater than normal."[25]

- *Deletion and "turning off" of genes:* Drs. Christopher Walsh and Eric Morrow of Harvard Medical School analyzed families in Middle East countries where there is a high incidence of autism and where there is an "increased tendency for cousins to marry, raising kids' odds of inheriting rare mutations." "The genetic analysis of these families revealed that autism is not only caused by the deletion of some genes but also by turning off other genes. These particular genes cause disruptions in the brain's ability to form new connections in response to experience."[26]

- *Observed genetic risk*: The highest risk factors in predicting AS are (1) blood ties (genes), someone else in the family is autistic; and (2) maleness.

Other Theories

- *Breakdown of the immune system:* "In children on the autistic spectrum assaults to the immune system could be occurring during the critical period of development in the second year of life when the body may not have enough vital force to fight infection and process touch, sound, sights, thoughts and feeling simultaneously. What would happen is the body puts all of its energy into staying alive. The immune system becomes hyper-vigilant and also irritable. This internal irritability can be observed outwardly as distractibility and hyperactivity, with development of sensory processing being severely retarded."[27]

- *Neanderthal Theory* claims that Asperger's Syndrome is caused by ancient hybridization of Neanderthals and Modern Man. Many of the traits and features of AS can be traced to the adaptive status of Neanderthals before the mutual mating. One example is the sensory system: "Sensory acuity varies widely between different species. Some species need very sensitive hearing, vision and smelling. These variations depend on the environment for which the animal is adapted. Neanderthals had adapted to a very different climate than modern humans. Therefore, it is likely there were sensory differences. Sensory differences are common in autistics. They can suffer from sensory overload by too sensitive senses but can also be very insensitive to certain types of pain."[28]

Geneticist Svante Paabo, at the Max Planck Institute for Evolutionary Anthropology in Leipzig, Germany, spearheaded a study that confirmed that modern humans in fact have Neanderthal genes. Colleagues identified small changes that are unique to human. "Some were in genes involved in energy metabolism, skeletal structure and brain development, including four that are thought to contribute to . . . autism, Down syndrome and schizophrenia."[29]

The shared genetic material could stem either from species hybridization or from a common ancestor.

- *Parents' genes in competition:* Two researchers, Dr. Bernard Crespi and Dr. Christopher Badcock, propose that "an evolutionary tug of war between genes from the father's sperm and the mother's egg can, in effect, tip brain development in one of two ways. A strong bias toward the father pushes a developing brain along the autistic spectrum toward a fascination with objects, patterns, mechanical systems, at the expense of social development. A bias toward the mother moves the growing brain along what the researchers call the psychotic spectrum, toward hypersensitivity to mood, their own and others." This "increases a child's risk of developing schizophrenia later on, as well as mood problems like bipolar disorder and depression."[30]

- *Extraterrestrial tinkering:* The theory of alien intervention stems from the idea often expressed by Aspies that they feel like aliens in this world. Could there have been interplanetary mating? Did aliens abduct and return earthlings after technologically manipulating genes?

Of course, considering our own Aspie son, Dylan, we could say that maybe, *after recognizing the genetic antecedents,* Dylan's "differences" *were* sparked by the spermicide use at conception, the prenatal electric shock or his lack of crawling as an infant.

Mirror Neurons

Countless hours of planned research into causes and effects have brought us only marginally closer to understanding the genesis of the autistic spectrum. However, we have been handed by way of accident a discovery that reveals what may be taking place neurologically in AS persons—the functioning of mirror neurons.

Neurophysiologists led by Giacomo Rizzolatti at the University of Parma, Italy, in the 1980s, stumbled upon the phenomenon. The scientists implanted electrodes in monkey brains to directly record neuron activity. They found that the same neurons are activated, or "fire," when a monkey either *performs* an action (say, picking up a piece of food), or when he *sees* another monkey perform the same action. Watching an action registered the same as performing an action! This is evidence of an emotional component; a connection from monkey to monkey, self to other, based on what a monkey only witnesses. Human brain activity measured by brain scan, though not as direct, is consistent with the monkey electrode finding and with findings in other primates.

This mirror-neuron concept recognizes the presence of specific neurons whose function is at the heart of social learning. The manner in which these mirror neurons function yields the most plausible explanation of "what is going on" neurologically to facilitate or impede a person in communicative learning. And it is this difference in neurology that accounts for behavioral differences between neurotypical and autistic spectrum persons.

The hypothesis for mirror-neuron activity in humans is that a neurotypical brain, *in addition* to simply seeing an action and being able to imitate another person's action, attaches *intent* and *emotional significance to the observed motion, which in turn gives that action context*. The viewer can then understand what the acting person is doing, feeling and intending. Through one's senses, the emotional state of the other person will be communicated. Consequently, a social tie, an understanding of the other person, is formed. "Grasping the emotional component of the various actions we observe around us is a crucial prerequisite for social communication. The skills needed to decode the emotional components of actions reach beyond the visuomotor representation of the observed movements. Additional perceptual and cognitive abilities are required to represent the emotional significance of the observed movements."[31] It is this *additional ability* that is the product of *typical* (NT) mirror-neuron activity. It is this ability that may be muted, distorted or misdirected in an *atypical* (AS) brain.

If the neural processing of observed action (movement) is at the crux of reading emotional components, we can say, then, that a person with *typically* functioning mirror neurons will view another person simply looking at an item of food and know that that person has intention of some sort regarding the food. (He witnessed the eye movement.) Furthermore, if the other person picks up the food, the observer will infer that the intention is to eat the food or at least do something further with it to satisfy an (emotional) need. The observer will frame both the eye movement toward the food and the movement of reaching for and picking it up in the context of the other person's *intention* to do something with the food item. Just by observing, a neurotypical person's neurons will fire; he will feel the same way the food-picker-upper feels, and he will get the significance, or *meaning*, of the other person's movements in the context of intention. He also probably will be able to predict that taking a bite of the food would likely follow in sequence; he would be surprised if the picker-upper stepped on or threw the apple. Once learned, the given movements related to an item that may be eaten are banked as a model in his brain: Looking at and picking up an item of food *means* the mover has a desire and intends to do something with the food to achieve an emotional goal (satisfaction.) He will have a context to predict other persons' behavior based on the model he has learned and incorporated.

If, however, a person with *atypically* functioning mirror neurons views the same scenario, he may not be able to interpret *intent* embodied in a person looking at or picking up the food. He can simply be a witness: a person looked at an apple, then picked up the apple then took a bite out of it. His observation is factual, he cannot "mind read," assigning the mental state or intention to the observed movement. He has no "saved" model for him to instantaneously grasp the significance or *meaning* of the motor action of looking at, then picking up a food item as precursor to the intention of eating to satisfy a need.

Correspondingly, he will not have a clue as to how anyone else (an NT) could tell that the item-picker-upper, simply by looking at food, had a plan for further action or for what that plan might be. Because persons in Aspiedom do not readily grasp *intention* in others, AS persons are often said to be "mind blind."

Our example using an item of food is *extremely* simplified for ease of exposition. In actuality, according to our mirror-neuron thesis, reading and interpretation of other persons' movements is a continuous neural function rather than isolated functions. Too, the system operates with regard to either large-motor action, such as seeing and interpreting the emotional state of someone running while glancing behind him, as well as to very small motor actions, including eye movement, facial expressions, posture, gestures, and other very subtle, involuntary body movements, such as pupil dilation and rate and depth of breathing. For the NT person, in the (social) presence of another person, with his mirror neurons firing, all movements of the other person contain a "readable" intentional/emotional element based on his internalized model of those actions.

Additionally, though the processing of *visuomotor* information is paramount to understanding context, other senses, such as hearing, must be similarly involved with mirror neurons. Do not most persons have an emotional reaction to *hearing* a car screech or someone yell? What if the sound of that car screech didn't register as someone else (emotionally) experiencing a roadway emergency or that someone yelling didn't signal some kind of emotional response in the hearing person? If one has *atypical* functioning mirror neurons and no way to place auditory stimuli into a context, how could he grasp the meaning? How could he translate that auditory information into feeling another person's experience?

Based on multiple sensory impressions, the functioning of mirror neurons can tell us why an NT person will be able to decode the very complex expression of, for example, crying, into subcategories. He will be able to translate even the small nuances of *why* another person cries. He can understand the contextual significance of both viewing and hearing a crying person and will recognize the composite subtleties that tell if that person is crying in pain, in sorrow, in relief, at frustration or anger, or at witnessing beauty. He will observe another person's tears and may be "moved" to tears himself—prima facie evidence that his mirror neurons have translated his sensory information into personal context.

Typical mirror-neuron activity is also confirmed as the NT person cheers up on seeing/hearing someone else laugh or winces when he sees someone trip and fall. He is scared when he sees and hears an angry person yell. He feels elation when his sports hero scores. He gets "turned on" when he watches a sexy movie . . . .

It is the parallel but *atypical* functioning of mirror neurons that is behind the AS person's lack of ability to recognize intentions and emotions of other persons. Predicting how another person will behave may be out of range. He may not intuitively understand the significance of seeing and hearing another person's emotional response. He simply may not recognize what another person feels, *unless that other person explicitly tells him*, or unless he has learned, by rote, the cues that signal particular emotions.

Unable to get information about feelings and mental states of other persons through body language, facial expression, vocal intonations, and other subtle nuances, he is dependent on the spoken word and pragmatic instruction to interpret and align his emotion to what he observes in others. Through no fault of his own, a person in Aspiedom cannot easily connect to another person with reciprocity of feeling, and he will have great difficulty learning the infinite intricacies of the social turf.

Because the Aspie does not thus easily *internalize* (social) models or boundaries of acceptable behavior, it is likewise difficult for him to appropriately frame his own actions and expressions. Consequently, continuing into adulthood, his behavior, body language, facial expression and speech may seem, in a vague way, "weird" or "odd."

Due to the fact that an AS person can't immediately identify the emotional state or intention of another person, he often is seen as someone who has no emotion himself. Make no mistake: The AS person *does* experience a deep well of emotion. He may have a difficult time either identifying or expressing his emotion. Just ask him about ardor for his interests or about yearning to 'fit in.' Without a doubt, he knows exactly the feelings of rejection and loneliness. He knows hurt, confusion, frustration, anger, depression, and hopelessness . . . .

Research and experimentation over the past thirty or so years indicates that natural genetic variation could account for Asperger's Syndrome, or that the genetic variation may be activated with single or multiple environmental factors. We can tag the immune system, prenatal insult, birth trauma, brain structures and connections. Causes may include Neanderthal genes, warring genes, or alien genes. And, we are impressed with the concept of mirror-neuron function as the most believable explanation of what is taking place neurologically in Asperger's Syndrome.

Once the AS person acquires some skill in reading emotional cues in other persons, he can compensate, to some degree, for his atypically responding mirror neurons. He can gradually develop socially as he learns how and when to respond "appropriately." He can work with nature's livery and with his fortune's star.

Until then, a person in Aspiedom stands apart, observing, analyzing, categorizing, and detailing the matter-of-fact world that his senses bring him . . . .

CRIME

"That it should come to this!"

—Hamlet

A typically developing teenager proactively seeks bonding with his peers. Social awareness increases, and the young adult develops a self-concept relative to his insight as an integral part of the social structure. He incorporates the standards and ethics of conduct from the outside in. He learns where behavioral boundaries are by interacting, communicating with other people. He learns intuitively from the reactions of other persons how he must behave *as well as* how he should not behave. He is a willing agent conforming to the culture's values to define himself as part of the collective.

An Aspie, too, will have a need to connect to his peers, but often will be confused about the how-tos of effective social and emotional function. He will not "pick up" on how others are feeling or learn from them appropriate responses. He simply does not easily learn how to "fit in." He will be cast by neurotypical, unaware schoolmates as an outsider, a weirdo, someone to exclude from their social circles.

As a result, the unidentified-as-Asperger's-Syndrome adolescent may become aware of his social ineffectiveness and his inability to make or sustain friendships. He will feel invisible or rejected by his peers. He will have no idea what is "wrong" with him. He may become depressed, anxious, frustrated, and withdrawn. Or he may act out in defiance, aggression, or verbal outbursts. According to Stephen Bauer, MD, MPH, "Pressure may build up . . . with little clue until he then reacts in a dramatically inappropriate manner."[1]

As the teenager progresses toward adulthood, he likely will learn some coping skills and may form friendships based primarily on common interests. However, socialization and behavioral adjustment complications probably will remain into adulthood. The AS person is on the periphery, with only a partially developed ability to recognize the timely behavioral norms, the social contracts. Because he cannot accurately interpret "the model," he does not know how the acceptable rules of behavior should interface with his own perceptions and emotions. He doesn't take the social pulse before speaking or acting. He cannot accurately measure the depth or breadth of his action in a social context; he is naive and may misunderstand. This debility, combined with low-impulse control, leaves the Aspie with a loose grip on his branch of the acceptable behavior tree. He may fall . . . .

Based on my day-to-day research, when an adult identified as an Asperger's Syndrome person has made headlines due to his maladaptive behavior, the following categories of criminal activity are the most likely: (1) hoax/impersonation/charade, (2) inappropriate (sexual) conduct, (3) fascination with chemical/incendiary processes, (4) cyber offenses, and (5) striking out at, especially stabbing, another person.

As might be expected, in no case did I discover any AS crime related to gangs (that would require interactive skills), robbery (planning, sequencing, interfacing), or exploitation and manipulation of others for personal gain. (An AS person would have difficulty even grasping the concept of exploiting others!)

As demonstrated in most of the following cases, an AS person will tell the truth. He will, in honesty and naivete, say, "I did it." If he makes the formal court plea "not guilty," it is because he is acting on the advice of an attorney, thereby being wedged into a legal system that does not appreciate honesty, but instead rewards whatever dishonesty one can get away with.

I list here synopses of cases that are of worldwide origin. Only crimes that *acknowledge* a role for Asperger's Syndrome or autism are included. I am *not*, in any way, suggesting that proportionately more or less crime is committed by AS persons than by members of the neurotypical population. In fact, Aspies are sometimes the *victims* of crimes because of their vulnerability to someone seeking to exploit them.

I include this chapter simply to help the reader grasp the fact that social violations happen because different neurologies render different perspectives on a given situation, and may well result in atypical actions/reactions.

Hoax/Impersonation/Charade

Nation: United Kingdom

Headline: "Teenager wings it with a fake airline"[2]

Synopsis: A seventeen-year-old convinced British aviation officials that he was launching a new airline. He posed as a visionary global entrepreneur and used phony websites to arrange a meeting with airport directors. He said he was in his twenties and he flew to Jersey to meet with the director of the airport. "Their talks were considered promising enough for a further meeting to be arranged."[2] They proposed to launch a cut-rate Channel Islands-based airline serving most of Europe. The ruse lasted six months while bogus articles were placed in industry magazines and floundered only after Airline World magazine became suspicious. The hoax unraveled as the network of fake websites was uncovered.

The teenager's father said his son suffered from a form of autism and "'was a phenomenal individual who is enterprising and creative,' with an ability to recall the exact detail of every airline's flight schedules."[2]

No further action was taken.

Nation: United Kingdom

Headline: "'Talented' Asperger's man escapes jail for exam fraud"[3]

Synopsis: A former banker and an economics student both pleaded guilty and were given suspended jail sentences for conspiracy to defraud the University of York. The student, who was "not particularly bright academically," asked the former banker, an Aspie, to take his exams for him and paid the Aspie to sit in his place using a false ID card in the student's name. The AS person's counsel said his Asperger's made him "vastly intelligent" but that it also could make him act in socially unacceptable ways. "He displays a genius but also displays a lack of insight in ordinary social norms." The judge said, "I'm persuaded that your underlying Asperger's condition has had a marked influence on your poor judgement as to what happened."[3]

Nation: United States

Headlines: "City's great train robber at it again: Serial subway impostor caught"[4]

"Transit Employee Impersonator Busted Again"[5]
"Avid Subway Enthusiast Arrested *Again*"[6]

Synopsis: A transit buff was arrested more than twenty times for impersonating a transit worker. The man was "collared for the first time at age 15 when he assumed the role and duties of a subway motorman, driving an E train full of passengers. "That was his best day that ever happened to him," said his mother."[5] More than 20 years later, he can't stay off the track."[4]

His most recent arrest came after he flashed a bogus badge and a forged ID card to a conductor after boarding a train. "Over the years he has donned MTA uniforms and cheerfully collected fares, cleared trash from tracks, put out underground fires."

Defenders of the now forty-three-year-old noted that he's never hurt anyone and that because of his Asperger's Syndrome his behavior reveals an "extreme preoccupation with a certain subject."[6]

Nation: Australia

Headline: "'Big cat handler' saved from the cage"[7]

Synopsis: To impersonate an employee, a nineteen-year-old man who "lives with Asperger Syndrome" had a uniform and vehicle made up to emulate those used at the zoo. "He took at least one couple on a tour of the zoo, pretending to be a big-cat handler and even taking them inside an enclosure . . . [His] charade extended to the Internet: a Wikipedia entry, which has been removed, listed him as one of the world's leading animal experts."[7]

Charges were dismissed on the condition that the defendant "not commit similar offences for a period of six months."

A neighbor said, "The young man had impersonated other professionals before and was known around town for being 'just like that kid from *Catch Me If You Can*, only better.'"[7]

Inappropriate Conduct

Nation: United States

Headline: "No jail sentence in child porn case"[8]

Synopsis: A twenty-one-year-old college student turned himself in and pleaded guilty to possessing child pornography. The judge was convinced that the defendant had "taken responsibility for the crime . . . and the problems behind it."[8] He was put on probation and had to register as a sex offender.

His attorney said the student had been diagnosed with Asperger's and that he was socially awkward. He also noted that his client took to the piano instantly at the age of 4: "The flip side of the gift of great talent is often a troubled existence in other aspects of one's life."[8]

Nation: United States

Headline: "Convicted N.J. Sex Offender to Get New Trial"[9]

Synopsis: New Jersey's highest court ruled that a new trial was in order so a sixty-two-year-old piano teacher previously convicted of molesting a young student could present expert testimony on his Asperger's diagnosis to explain his conduct. He wanted to show the jury why he may make inappropriate social judgments.

In the original trial, the prosecution had said that by pulling a female student onto his lap and touching her over her clothing he was "grooming her for future sexual assault by familiarizing her with such contact."[9]

The Asperger's expert stated that "persons with [AS] generally do not have the ability to manipulate people easily because of their weakness in detecting social cues that other persons readily recognize."[9]

Nation: United Kingdom

Headline: "'Terrible Twins' given ASBOs"[10] [Anti Social Behavior Orders]

Synopsis: "Young tearaways," twenty-year-old girls, "threatened, abused and ridiculed" neighborhood residents. The pair's lawyers said, "The twins suffered from Asperger's Syndrome, which meant they would have difficulties in understanding and complying properly with the ASBO."[10]

A consulting psychiatrist said, "Their condition meant they could understand the ASBO conditions but they had difficulties comprehending the impact of breaking them.

"She also said they were liable to act impulsively, without any thoughts about the consequences of their actions."[10]

Nation: United States

Headline: "The Physicist and the Torched SUVs"[11]

Synopsis: A twenty-four-year-old "brilliant but quirky physics grad student"[11] faced trial on federal arson counts.

With two others, the student was charged with torching 14 Hummers and a building, claiming responsibility in the name of Earth Liberation Front. The defendant said he never committed arson, but he didn't deny being present that night. His lawyers explained the apparent contradiction by "showing that (their client) has Asperger's Syndrome, a mild form of autism marked by an impaired ability to comprehend social situations. The question is: how can somebody so smart be so dumb? . . . Asperger's answers that question."[11]

His behavior was described as particularly odd because he put the FBI on his trail by writing an arcane equation on one of the SUVs, then writing about it in an e-mail traced to a university computer.

He was sentenced to eight years in federal prison for conspiracy to commit arson. The arson conviction was overturned on appeal (the omission of the Asperger Syndrome diagnosis during the original trial played a role in the overturned decision) but the conspiracy conviction was upheld. The prisoner is to be released in August 2011.

Nation: United Kingdom

Headline: "Drug dealer 'acting like a child'"[12]

Synopsis: A twenty-two-year-old man was accused of buying drugs with the intent to sell them. His defense attorney argued that his client had been diagnosed with Asperger's Syndrome and "is essentially operating at the level of a young child."

The accused, the attorney said, "had bought the drugs because he thought it would enhance his status." He also noted that the man had paid more for the drugs than they were worth.[12]

The defendant was sentenced to 120 hours of community service and ordered to return before the court so his progress could be evaluated.

Nation: United States

Headline: "Conn. teen with autism held in assault rifle shooting"[13]

Synopsis: A sixteen-year-old boy with Asperger's Syndrome approached a group of young men playing basketball. The ball bounced off the rim and hit the teenager, who became angry.

He began to talk of having a gun, and started to pick a fight with one of the young men, said a member of the group. "One of my friends told him to get out of here and called him an 'idiot.'"[13] The group laughed about the gun threat.

The teen left angry, then returned with an assault rifle. He told the group not to come closer. "I don't want to shoot you."[13] He turned the rifle to the sky and fired a shot. One young man wrestled the teen to the ground and another shot went off. The group of friends started punching the teen in the face, freed the gun and held him on the ground until police arrived. No one was injured.

The teen's father said his son's condition is characterized by eccentric behavior. "Any slight you give a kid with Asperger's, it's magnified 10 times . . . then, if they feel threatened, it's 10 times more . . . It can become a powder keg."[13]

Nation: United Kingdom

Headline: "Teen fired BB gun at folk for fun"[14]

Synopsis: An eighteen-year-old man was reported to police after he fired his BB gun at a mother pushing her two-year-old along a road. He "happily admitted he was firing the weapon out of the window at people" ... and that he was doing it for the fun of it.

The court deferred sentence after hearing that the teenager "suffered from various symptoms of Asperger's syndrome and obsessive compulsive behavior."[14]

Nation: Australia

Headline: "Family takes revenge on sex attacker"[15]

Synopsis: A twenty-seven-year-old diagnosed with Asperger's Syndrome and attention deficit disorder met teens aged 13 and 15 through an Internet chat room. He subsequently engaged in sexual acts with them. He was abducted, bashed, interrogated and threatened with death by a relative of one of the victims before he was handed over to police.

He did not make a complaint against the family because he "thought he might have got what he deserved."[15] His father told the court that "his son was a very lonely young man who had a level of maturity very low for his age."[15]

The court psychiatrist gave evidence that the defendant was not intellectually aware of the age of consent and "did not have a systematic way for working out what was right or wrong."[15]

The defendant pled guilty to nine charges. No sentencing information was available.

Nation: United States

Headline: "Autistic man to live under supervision after child enticement charge"[16]

Synopsis: A twenty-three-year-old man was accused of attempting to entice a four-year-old boy. He said that "he liked playing with kids and he has no friends his own age."[16] Court documents said the man has Asperger's Syndrome. "Characteristics of the disorder include socially and emotionally inappropriate behavior, the inability to interact successfully with peers, peculiarities in speech and language, and obsessive interest in narrow topics . . ."[16]

He was found "not guilty by reason of mental disease or defect."[16]

Fascination with Chemical/Incendiary Processes
Nation: Australia

Headline: "Chemistry fan jailed over drug haul"[17]

Synopsis: A thirty-five-year-old man pleaded guilty to trafficking in a large commercial quantity of methamphetamine from a backyard laboratory. Police described the operation as "sophisticated."

The judge said the manufacturer, "who studied part of a science degree majoring in chemistry, had an IQ in 'the very superior range' and suffered Asperger's syndrome . . . He was obsessed with chemical processes, and making drugs provided an outlet for him.'"[17]

He was sentenced to fifteen years and three months jail.

Nation: United Kingdom

Headlines: "Bomb-making teenager could be sectioned"[18]
"Medical order on shed 'bombmaker'"[19]

Synopsis: A nineteen-year-old with a recent diagnosis of Asperger's Syndrome was charged with making explosives—"bangers"—in a backyard shed. "We knew he was mixing things in the shed," said the teen's father. "We shouldn't have let him piddle around with that stuff... He was just making those bangers, but these were really big ones."[18]

"There was no question of criminal or terrorist intent," said the prosecutor. "The defendant clearly has a fascination with explosions. He started doing it to give his air gun more thrust."[19]

The judge imposed a two-year community order with a mental health requirement.

Nation: United States:

Headline: "Bombs net man 5 years' probation"[20]

Synopsis: A twenty-year-old man avoided prison time for manufacturing bombs because he suffers from a "mental disorder that borders on autism."[20]

The judge believed that the man never intended to harm anyone and concluded that probation would be the best way to salvage the defendant so that he could be a productive member of society.[20]

Cyber Offense

Nation: New Zealand

Headline: "Alleged cyber crime kingpin suffers autism"[21]

Synopsis: An eighteen-year-old who left school in year 9, then continued with correspondence school, is the suspected "AKILL," the cyber ringleader of a "botnet" that has infected a million computers with a virus resulting in major economic loss.

Friends and employers praised the young man as a brilliant computer programmer. The manager of the police national electronic crime laboratory said the youth was "very, very bright in terms of his ability to be able to produce that sort of code."[21]

The teenager lost his job as a programmer, but the company director said that the teen did not actively seek trouble or illegal activity.

Nation: United Kingdom/United States

Headlines: "British computer hacker faces extradition to US after court appeal fails"[22]

"[Suspect's] mother to Obama: Please Help!"[23]

Synopsis: A forty-two-year-old man has been described in the United States as "the biggest military hacker of all time"[22] and faces charges of breaking into U.S. Army, Navy, and NASA computer systems, admittedly looking to "discover the truth about what he believed was the coverup of information on UFOs, reverse engineering, Free energy and anti gravity."[23]

The man was arrested in the UK. For seven years, U.S. authorities have been trying to extradite him to stand trial.

The suspect "has always been naive and young for his age, which I [his mother] now realize is part and parcel of his Asperger's syndrome. A requirement of Asperger's is intelligence and Aspies usually have a heightened sense of justice. He also tells the truth even to his own detriment."[23] "[An AS person's] passions become obsessions followed through with a single-minded tunnel vision that often lands people with Asperger's in trouble."[23]

As *WWDYM* manuscript goes to print, the case is not yet resolved.

Striking Out at Another Person

Nation: Japan

Headlines: "Man jailed for 26 years for fatal knife attack on group of laughing students"[24]
"Manslaughter conviction after stabbing"[25]

Synopsis: A twenty-two-year-old man was convicted of attacking a group of five high school students who were laughing near his home. One student died and another was seriously injured.

The defendant admitted to the charges from the outset. A psychiatric evaluation used in court said that he had Asperger's Syndrome, rendering his ability to control his actions weak. The group of laughing students revived memories of unpleasant experiences when he was teased in school, prompting him to attack.

[The defendant's] defense had argued his mental competency was diminished at the time of the attack but the court rejected the argument. He was sentenced to twenty-six years behind bars.[24]

Nation: Australia

Headlines: "Killer had autistic disorder: court"[26]
"Judge rules [defendant] didn't murder mother"[27]

Synopsis: A twenty-three-year-old man admitted fatally stabbing his mother after she and he argued and she threatened him with a knife to "get out or she would call the police . . ."[26] The court psychiatrist said the defendant had symptoms consistent with Asperger's Syndrome, and therefore "was unable to understand social norms or nuances in conversation, his speech was 'monotone, almost robotic' and he had obsessional interests." He also informed the court that "people with Asperger's typically had an inability to understand other people's thoughts and feelings." The prosecution "has to prove the defendant intended to kill his mother or was 'recklessly indifferent' to whether his actions would kill her."[26]

The defendant was found not guilty of murdering his mother, but was convicted instead of manslaughter.[27]

Nation: United Kingdom

Headline: "Stepson stabbed woman to death"[28]

Synopsis: A twenty-one-year-old man told his aunt, in a telephone conversation, that he had stabbed his stepmother. "He kept saying he was sorry and that he loved me." The police came while the alleged assailant was on the phone and his aunt "kept telling him he must tell them he had Asperger's." She wanted the police to know because she was concerned about how they would deal with him. "He would not like to be handled or restrained."[28]

In an earlier call the same day, the defendant told his aunt his "dad was an idiot and had been starting on him in the pub and had then gone off and left him."[28] The defendant denied murder on the grounds of diminished responsibility.

He was convicted of manslaughter.

Nation: United States

Headlines: "Wife-slaying Linux guru may have 'developmental disability'"[29]

"Reiser Found Guilty of Missing Wife's Murder"[30]
"Reiser found guilty of first degree murder"[31]

Synopsis: A forty-four-year-old academic prodigy who entered college at age fourteen, became a software programmer and developed the ReiserFS file system was accused of murdering his wife. The defending attorney said that "the defendant may be mentally incompetent as a result of mental disorder or developmental disability."[29] He suffers from a form of autism called Asperger's Disorder and that the "condition explained why he doesn't behave well in social settings and acted strangely after [his wife] disappeared"[30] A systems competitor said the defendant was "a talented programmer whose work was overshadowed by his temperament... He was not the easiest person to work with... He was technically brilliant but socially not at quite the same level."[31]

The defendant was sentenced, then led police to his wife's buried body and subsequently received a reduction in the possible twenty-five-year jail sentence.

As Asperger's Syndrome is only a very recent diagnosis, all of these headlines are likewise recent. This does not negate the idea that court cases have come and gone for years, or are pending at this time, with unidentified AS persons as defendants.

Asperger's Syndrome does not necessarily free one from culpability, but it may mitigate the responsibility. The increasing awareness of the role that the autistic spectrum plays in society throws the court system some extraordinary new challenges. How does the legal system handle an alleged perpetrator's fragile sense of social impact? Does the AS person's lack of judgment translate as diminished capacity? Instead of decreased *mental* capacity, might a new defense be a decreased *social* capacity? Just how "willful" is the offense? Is there a degree of malice or intent? How much? Was the accused just curious about what would happen if he did X, Y, or Z without taking notice of social significance? Can a motive be accurately asserted?

While researching this chapter, reading *The Psychiatric Times* newsletter, I came across the following standard that psychiatrists use to determine the *treatment capacity* of a patient. I was struck by a synchronous idea that the same criteria may be appropriate for our courts to determine the *social capacity of* an Asperger's Syndrome person when charged with a crime: "(1) the ability to understand relevant information, (2) the ability to appreciate the situation and its consequences, (3) the ability to manipulate the relevant information rationally, and, (4) the ability to express a stable, voluntary choice."[32] Perhaps it will come to this . . .

ASPIES SPEAK

"This above all: to thine own self be true."

—Hamlet

The best way for a neurotypical person to understand Asperger's Syndrome is to read the writings of AS persons, to themselves being true. Though we've established AS persons *will* have impairment in *reciprocal* conversation, in nonverbal communication, and in processing spoken language, their written language skills often are well developed. And as seen through several Internet forums and blogs, they do want to share, to have community.

Disclaimer: I have no way to verify the Aspie validity of any of these entries. Likewise, I have no reason to doubt any of them. I have included the ages of the posters where available and, because this book is about adults, have not quoted anyone with a listed age of less than eighteen years.

On Processing Spoken Language
("Wait, What Do You Mean?")

Eileen Parker, a.k.a. cozycalm: "Only so much input at once, is my rule. So, say the bare bones of what you have to say, then stop—unless you are communicating with facial expressions, tones of voice, and hand gestures. Then you will have to state those unvoiced messages because I didn't receive them. They are visual distortion of the message."[1]

FJ Stout, a.k.a. Fiz: "I cannot work with high volumes of people that are always different, i.e. customers, as most people are rude and tough to talk to and I don't always understand what they are asking for."[2]

bettybarton (age 35): "In fact, I just have problems listening sometimes, and following verbal instructions."[3]

aphonos (age 28): "I think that the child-like nature of my speech is caused by the stress and confusion of real-time conversation. I become very anxious knowing that someone is expecting a response immediately as this does not give me time to process what they have said or to translate my reply into something they can understand."[4]

Lynne Soraya: "The brain in a person with AS is similar to a computer which has a huge hard drive but with a slow audio and video processor and not enough RAM. So like the computer can lock up when it has inadequate resources to manage incoming data, so does the AS brain when too much is going on. You get 'memory overflow' when there isn't enough room in the buffer to save the incoming data until it gets permanently saved on the hard drive, so data is lost."[5]

Adrian, a.k.a. AS-4-L: "When there are a lot of sounds going on, it's like they all have the same volume. I can't tune in or tune out to any one sound.

"This makes it so hard to participate in group conversations that you start to not bother . . . Frustration and overload set in and you retreat into yourself. . . . It's not that I have nothing to say, it's just that I can't navigate this auditory environment. I can't pick and find my way; it's an assault course for which I have no answer. When you've finally thrown in the towel you just sit and stare into space while others converse around you. You then start to realize that you don't really want to talk to these people anyway, you're only trying to fit in and do what they do. That is the moment of no return."[6]

Emoal6: "Aspies are usually very intelligent, they can just lack an ability to formulate their opinions and knowledge in a socially acceptable way.

"It is hard for us to speak in person or on the phone even. We hear too much around us, we get walked over in conversations or do the opposite. Writing is just the preferred form of communication because it shows dedication to our thought. It also doesn't allow you to interrupt and throw us off course, or of what we meant to say."[7]

miniMAX: "Following threads of conversations is the hardest. I'm a non-stop series of non-sequiturs."[8]

Nonliteral language: It is frequently stated in the literature that Aspies cannot "get" sarcasm, metaphors, jokes, *nonliteral* language, and body language. Here are some Aspie takes on these particular forms of expression:

Tracker (age 21): "[I have] some trouble with non-literal language. (I do fine with this when I can see it coming. For example, when I watch the Daily Show, I expect there to be sarcasm, so I am not confused by it. Likewise I don't have a problem with metaphor in poetry because I expect it to be there. But in [conversation] sarcasm/metaphor/innuendo I have trouble picking it up.)"[9]

Sedaka (age 26): "I use metaphors, etc. fine . . . though I've heard them all before and I get them . . . and I do still get tripped up over other ones in conversation from time to time. Point is, you're not stupid. . . . You can learn what is meant by the expression and then use it.

"And I will say, that the times that I do have troubles with them is usually when people are joking about something and are alluding to some unknown thing . . . If I don't even know what we're talking about, then I'm probably not even going to recognize the metaphor."[10]

Danielismyname: "It generally means that you may have trouble with understanding metaphors that aren't familiar to you, when people say that those with AS may have problems with 'metaphors.' It doesn't mean that you can't use them."[11]

Susan Jaye Graham, a.k.a. sartresue: "When I hear . . . a metaphorical expression for the first time I get a literal picture of it and then I decipher it. So my learning is slower than an NT. When I heard the expression, 'One swallow does not make a summer,' I asked what was meant by the word 'swallow.' When told this was a sort of bird I imagined a sea gull flying by itself. Then I asked why one swallow does not make a summer and was told that just because you see one swallow flying around this does not mean summer is here yet. I then imagined a whole sky full of these birds being needed before the season of summer officially started. The larger meaning I was told was that one should never jump to conclusions. This made sense. More proof is needed before concluding a rule. This is logic. But I still see the swallow(s) when someone mentions this expression. It would seem to indicate that somewhere along the line someone talked about birds and whether seeing one was a harbinger of summer. I wonder what sort of avian species is associated with autumn?"[12]

Angela, a.k.a. Ticker: "Actually I've seen speaking in metaphors as a symptom of Asperger's. Some severe Aspies can only converse that way as they are unable to come up with their own original words."[13]

hiccup: "I often memorize phrases that people use to say certain things, so I can use them to say the same thing, but can't fully understand the meaning enough to generalize the usage for purposes or conversations outside of the purpose for which I've memorized the phrase/word."[14]

And curious myself about (English major) Dylan's ability to understand metaphors, I challenged him while talking with him on the phone: "What does it mean when people use the expression, 'When pigs fly?'" Without hesitation, he responded, "Is that like when hell freezes over?" Bingo! My delight in his answer using a metaphor to explain a metaphor and a question to answer my question was obvious in my laughter, prompting him to state (using a simile!) that he felt like he "just won a contest!" (See **POSTSCRIPT**) Answering a question with a question is a developed form of **echoalia**, or bounce-back communication, another Aspie trait and one that Dylan often uses. Of the forty or so other adults that I subsequently queried, all but one explained the "when pigs fly" metaphor with the nonmetaphor, "It's not going to happen." Only one other person responded as Dylan did, with another metaphor, "It'll be a cold day in hell." Keeping it in the family, that person was Dylan's uncle, my brother.

On How to Get a Diagnosis

donkey: "There are no definitive diagnostic tests for AS. There are DSM-IV criteria but it is all subjective and different countries have different criteria for a formal diagnostic approach.

"Warning: for every psychologist that is legitimate there will be 100 other 'paraprofessionals' who are willing to take your money at your time of anxiety: dietitians, speech therapists, psychologists and psychiatrists, heavy metal testing, brain scanning testing, music teaching therapists, interventionists who want to cure ASD's, clothing manufacturers who will sell you ASD clothing, animal therapists who offer ASD's friendly horses and monkeys . . . life coaches, ASD consultants, frustrated mothers groups . . . everything and everyone will tell you that their method is better and is worth paying for while criticizing the other.

"My advice: see a psychologist (not a psychiatrist) who specializes in ASD's. Develop a relationship with them and take their advice, but be aware the psychologist will be under pressure to refer you to others who want a slice of the AS action. It's a new and growing cottage industry surrounding ASD's that is growing and exploiting the lack of an objective definitive test and diagnosis for ASD's. Why take my advice? I'm 37, I'm AS, my son is 6 and AS. I have seen them all. But most importantly . . . my advice is free!"[15]

On Diagnostic Difficulty

Because Asperger's Syndrome has been identified and regarded as a diagnosis in psychiatric literature only for the past few years, practicing physicians and psychotherapists who trained *prior* to AS recognition may have no education on this neurology. Asperger's Syndrome, therefore, may not even be included in their diagnostic vocabulary. Furthermore, many diagnosticians in the mental health field are not as familiar with *developmental* disorders as they are with *behavioral* disorders and therefore diagnose solely within *behavioral* parameters.

This means that an adult displaying the *behaviors* of compulsiveness, anxiety, depression, and poor impulse control may be diagnosed as having **O**bsessive-**C**ompulsive **D**isorder, Social Anxiety, **B**ipolar **D**isorder, **ADD**, **ADHD**, or **D**epression. However, these individual diagnoses may *together* be part of the package of traits that coexist with the single, *developmental* condition of **A**sperger's **S**yndrome.

As social awareness of the need to address AS adults increases, the availability of qualified specialists who *can* accurately identify or diagnose will correspondingly increase. We can look forward to better professional services to accurately identify adults or to validate the identity of self-suspected Asperger's Syndrome persons.

But until that happens, Gyasi Burks-Abbot, Aspergers Association of New England board member, says many Aspie adults can end up with an "Asperger's pedigree" of this, that, and other diagnoses received before "stumbling on Asperger's Syndrome!" To wit:

sem1precious (age 32): "I have Asperger's but I haven't been diagnosed yet . . . I have just about every diagnosis that if they just lumped them all together it would be Asperger's but for some reason, they keep trying to talk me out of it.

"Here's what I have so far: Generalized Anxiety Disorder, Panic Attacks, Chronic Depression, 'over focused' ADD, flat affect, and sensory issues. But I think that because I can 'talk' to them, that they think I'm OK, or something. However, if they were to put me in a room with two or three of them, they would be able to see my problems very obviously. I can seem to be normal when talking one on one, but any more and I get lost very easily. I can also only handle 'acting normal' for short periods of time, during which I experience increasing levels of anxiety."[16]

ngonz (age 50): "Most medical professionals in [Wisconsin] don't know anything about autism or Asperger's. Some have never even heard the term Asperger's and have asked me what it is and how to spell it. Sheesh!"[17]

GodsWonder: "I went for diagnosis a few days ago expecting to be diagnosed with Asperger's Syndrome because I have the majority of the symptoms, rather I was just diagnosed with the general PDD-NOS. I am supposed to go back for a final evaluation and diagnosis soon but I feel that the psychiatrist does not know exactly what he is talking about. The psychiatrist evaluated me for Asperger's and he agreed that I had most of the symptoms. He then asked me if I get lonely and have a desire to make friends and I said yes. He then said that he thinks that I might have something other than Asperger's because people with Asperger's don't want to have friends and that they don't have any desire for friends and he said he thinks I have either avoidant personality disorder or social anxiety. I agree that I have social anxiety disorder but only as a result of my social awkwardness from Asperger's. I had researched avoidant personality disorder and people with that disorder are more likely to not want friends than people with Asperger's because they are afraid of people criticizing them. Also, I didn't have the majority of the symptoms that come with avoidant personality disorder."[18]

craola: "It doesn't make sense, but most psychiatrists really shouldn't be diagnosing Autistic Spectrum Disorders. It's not what they are trained for and they don't understand the full scope of what it incorporates. My psych, when I first told him what my psychologist and I had been talking about the AS, he said no, no way because I wasn't like the *Rain Man*. Of the three I've had none have been clued up about it. Specialists are always best it seems."[19]

obnoxiously-me (age 32): "I don't have an official Aspie or like diagnosis, as I'm tired of seeing psychiatrists and their pills. I have been diagnosed:
Schizoid Personality Disorder
Schizo-affective
OCD [Obsessive Compulsive Disorder]

PTSD [Post Traumatic Stress Syndrome]
Depression
Borderline pd [personality disorder?]
Schizophrenia
Anxiety
Non 24-hour sleep disorder
And the nice 'multi (split or whatever) personality' one too. Nice bag of crackers. Crunch.
They put me on medication, and that just gets worse. Then I become psychotic, especially on the anti depression medication."[20]

Who_Am_I (age 33): "This isn't a diagnosis, but my psychiatrist keeps mentioning 'avoidant behavior.' I wish he'd learn the difference between avoidant behavior and having a brain with a faulty 'start' button."[21]

BrixBrix: "I'm like 99.9% sure I have it. My mom and I went to a psychologist about it and after less than 10 minutes, my mom asked the doc if I had it. The doc laughed in our faces and simply said I was too smart to have it and completely threw it out as a diagnostic possibility. (Keep in mind this is only after 10 mins). She's apparently got no experience with Asperger's because she should know that ppl [people] with it have above average intelligence. So instead of one diagnosis, the doc diagnosed me with a crapload of anxiety and sensory disorders as well as depression. All of the things I was diagnosed with are little pieces of Aspergers. It's like my doc wasn't looking at the whole picture.

"I'm wondering if I should go to another doctor. One who has experience with Aspergers. Because here are my symptoms:

- No friends
- Never had serious b/f [best friend]

- Monotone voice
- Lack empathy
- Have to have routine
- Depression
- Extreme anxiety daily
- Hate being around ppl
- Don't understand ppl
- Very OCD (have been clinically diagnosed with it as well)
- Repetitive movements
- Can't make eye contact
- Absolute pitch (can hear a music note and name it instantly)
- Clumsy
- Have to wear earplugs in public and at school
- Sensory problems
- Very ritualistic, do same things same way each time in same order
- Extremely obsessive
- Problems processing auditory information
- Often echo what people say without conscious effort

"And I honestly don't know how in the hell my psychologist can overlook all that and diagnose me with a bunch of small disorders instead of one bigger one."[22]

flamingshorts: "I've been diagnosed with depression, hypomania, 'he's just shy,' social anxiety disorder, etc. Now at the age of 47 finally get Asperger's or maybe PDD-NOS. Even then I had to 'suggest' the diagnosis to my psychiatrist who agreed."[23]

Angnix (age 26): "I currently have the horrible label of Schizoaffective Disorder. I am for sure Bipolar and my medications are actually for

Bipolar and work well, but I am missing the vast majority of schizophrenia symptoms ... And my psychologist ignores my Aspie-like symptoms ... probably because I'm female, but I don't know if I'm really Aspie or just eccentric with weird motor mannerisms and no social skills."[24]

Vimse (age 31): "Borderline personality disorder, bipolar disorder, schizoaffective disorder and schizophrenia. Mental health professionals don't seem to know what they are doing. Luckily all of these diagnoses were removed when my autism was discovered."[25]

And prior to there being any recognition of AS, some persons were sent to psychiatric hospitals and labeled with a multitude of *recognized* mental illnesses.

John Harold, writing a profile in the Papakura Courier: "Jen had struggled for more than 40 years with undiagnosed Asperger Syndrome and had spent months at Kingseat psychiatric hospital.

"Doctors tried in vain to help Jen and pondered whether she was suffering from schizophrenia, borderline personality disorder, manic depression, anxiety disorder for the beginning stages of multiple personality disorder."[26]

On Identification as an AS person

Rebecca_L (age 45): "Last year my 4 1/2 year old grandson was diagnosed with Autism. While researching it ... I came across the description of Asperger's ... There was an instant 'That's ME!' as I read it."[27]

hiccup: "Hey. I think I am Asperger's. I am almost positive. I can't believe it's taken so long to figure it out. My life has sucked so much and I always thought I was just some freak."[28]

Willard: "Since Asperger Syndrome wasn't even on the psychological radar until '94, more and more adults every day are discovering... the cause behind all those quirks we used to think were just our own personal deficiencies. I'm 49 and only heard of AS for the first time about four years ago."[29]

Vanilla_Slice: "Ah!! All of a sudden we discovered the reason why everything had been going wrong for the last twenty or thirty years. My only regret is that AS hadn't been recognized in the mid 1970s when, in my case, it all started going pear shaped."[30]

flamingshorts: "Since self-diagnosing Asperger's I haven't had depression, I've had hope. Frustration too, but hope."[31]

Aysmptotes: "I found out that I had AS through a Youtube video when I was nineteen. After that . . . I read quite a few things on AS, a few books and articles. At first it kind of floored me and I felt this huge relief that it all wasn't my fault and that this is just how I am."[32]

Reclusive: "I was diagnosed with Asperger's Syndrome quite late on in my life, at the age of 42. This was after many years of depression and after a lifetime of knowing that I was not like other people. I never fitted in anywhere, ever since I started school I had felt very abnormal and had always sensed that there was something very 'wrong' with me, but I just didn't know what it was."[33]

Jael: "I am 44 years old and you can't imagine how it feels to find out at this age why it is that I am so fundamentally different from everyone I know. THIS is why I express myself in formal language that makes me sound as though I stepped out of the 18th century! THIS is why I am so often obsessive about things that interest me. And most of all, THIS is why normal social interaction has always been impossibly difficult for me! There's actually a NAME for this!"[34]

Alyson Bradley: "I have spent a whole lifetime being on the outside and so badly wanting to come in, but never knew how until now. Before it was like being in a time capsule, but I broke out and made sense of Asperger's and found my real self.

"I now feel like at last I have been saved, but would not wish my journey on anyone, it's been far too hard and painful at times. No one really seemed to understand, believe in or has been willing to let me simply be me. Growing up and not knowing is a bit like being wrongly imprisoned."[35]

WonderWoman: "I'm 55 and to find out that there are others learning to cope with this. Wow!"[36]

Julie Langdale: "Being diagnosed was the single most cathartic moment in my life and I feel that more people need to step forward, stand up, and say 'I Exist.'"[37]

Stew54: "Finding out about AS has been an absolute revelation. It explains me to myself so much better than anything ever has before, and that's enough for me."[38]

Charles Pierce: "At the age of 60 I was told by two qualified people who have known me for decades, that I have Asperger's Syndrome. This information was a revelation and a liberation. The course of my life was explained, not excused, but explained, and a clear road to future progress opened up."[39]

Silke: "I came to consider Asperger's after a long time researching all sorts of disorders based on the odd behaviors I have and always had. OCD, social anxiety, tics . . . it was all there but I had looked at them as separate issues. Then I came across the description for Asperger's and something clicked. I ticked all the boxes and suddenly everything made sense. Why I find it so hard to look people in the eyes. Why honesty and fairness is such a big issue. Why I find it so hard to connect to my 'peers' and could never understand 'small talk.' Why I am so clumsy. Why I love solitude and retreating into my own head. Why I'm so tense and anxious. Why I can't grieve. Why I'm so sensitive to loud noises. Why I fall to pieces at the smallest bit of criticism . . . the list goes on and on.

"Once I connected the dots and came to the Aspie conclusion there was a certain calm in my head. I guess having found a plausible explanation has removed a lot of the uncertainty and fear about myself. I have stopped beating myself up about my failure to connect and am less hard on myself."[40]

Linda Jones, a.k.a. earthmom: "I'm a 47 year old Aspie and I've hidden my quirks as much as possible all of my life.

"Four years ago I started evolving—that's the only word for it—dropping the pretenses. I learned about Asperger's. I read a lot and learned and was thrilled to have this answer finally."[41]

Sheila Schoonmaker: "Before knowing about Asperger's, I endlessly tried to find a way to fit in with the world somehow. I thought I couldn't exist until someone would let me in to validate me. The way I craved to be let in was for someone to share the mysteries that everyone else but me seemed to know. I'd describe it as being like the solitary child who the others won't let join their club house."[42]

Linda Jones, a.k.a. earthmom: "If the 'norm' was all a flock of birds and I was an elephant, I would spend my life hearing 'She's too big. She needs to be smaller.' 'Her beak is too long—she should have that changed.' 'Why is she that color? Gray is awful—she needs to buy some products to become this nice shade of yellow like the rest of us' and I'm flapping my legs and trying to make bird sounds and never accomplishing the goal until one day I meet a herd of elephants. OMG!

"Then I realize—I'm not a BAD BIRD, I'm a GREAT ELEPHANT! I don't have to change and try to be that—I'm a whole 'nuther' species and there are a LOT of us!

"Such celebration! Such freedom!

"That's how I felt learning about AS."[43]

Athena Franks: "I have always felt like the odd one out, and often was reprimanded for my behavior as a child. Often an outcast. When I was a young adult I found out about Asperger's Syndrome . . . and it was like a light went on in my dark universe. I finally had some context for what had marked me."[44]

Acacia: "The thing is I had no idea about Asperger's until about two months ago. When I suddenly saw how it explained my entire life, I knew that I had it."[45]

AC132: "I saw a documentary on AS that dropped my jaw and made me weep with that [AS] realization. My whole life made sense in that moment. My *whole* life."[46]

Pragmaticus: "When I was 16 years old, I was diagnosed with Asperger's Syndrome. In short, it answered all my questions. My analogy is this: most computers come with their software pre-installed. Most people are born with their social software already built in. People with Asperger's, however, have to install their social software manually."[47]

Pat (age 21): "At first it was a shock, and it made me cry because I lost hope of ever falling in love, holding a job, meeting new friends, etc. But now it feels like since I know what I have, I can take advantage of it (my Asperger's) . . . Since learning that I have Asperger's, I have been trying to think more positively and I've been listening to more positive music."[48]

Tim Gilbert, a.k.a. glider18: "I was diagnosed with Asperger's as an adult. It hasn't bothered me any. If anything, it has helped me. I have finally found who I am—and I am still getting to know myself. I find it quite fascinating.

"I had received a diagnosis that showed how my life fit together sensibly . . . No longer do I worry about my eccentric ways—I am proud of them."[49]

vulcanpastor: "I got my diagnosis today: I do have Asperger's. It's kind of a relief. After years of not fitting in and feeling like a failure, I now have a language to explain who I am."[50]

On Post Identification Adjustment

Sheila Schoonmaker: "For a very brief time after learning that the 'gap' was due to a neurological difference between me and the majority of others, I felt sad over knowing that it was time for me to let go of the hope I'd been clinging to throughout my life. Once I accepted this loss, I was stunned to discover a joy I'd never have thought possible for me to experience. That joy came from knowing that there never really was anything 'wrong' with me after all! It was merely an illusion I allowed others to place upon me."[51]

Aspie Speaks about Aspie Children

Roger J. Balogh, MD (Dr. Balogh is a psychiatrist who was diagnosed with Asperger's Syndrome at age fifty-two): "Early in life, many of these children appear strange and unusual. In a sense these children have a mind which operates lake a race car with no instructions on how to drive it. They take off and crash repeatedly. Messages may go to the wrong part of the brain. Messages may get reversed, inverted or jumbled. Thoughts may have trouble being converted into actions. All aspects of sensory and motor function may, to some degree, be involved. Their world is very chaotic and confusing. The experience is, to say the least, overwhelming. The result is high levels of anxiety and frustration which culminate in emotional outbursts or shutting down. In order to control this chaos, a child resists change in his environment. They will repeat the behavior for as long as it takes for the anxiety to resolve."[52]

On Experience as an Aspie

Jeffery Serio, a.k.a. Abstract_Logic (age 21): "I am not insane, I am not sane, either. I am just juxtaposed to the prejudice of what people so inaptly refer to as 'normal.'"[53]

Adrian, a.k.a. AS-4-L: "Having AS is having a frustrating, scary, and at times hard to deal with life. We often get overloaded and just fail at being able to cope. When I find myself in those lowest of times I do self-harm. I cut myself and have in the past (but only as a never-repeated experiment) burned myself. I've done other things that I'll stop short of telling you about, but needless to say my body is a patchwork of history."[54]

Tracker (age 21): "I always knew that I was different, even from my first days in school. But I had always assumed that my problems (bad handwriting, trouble recognizing faces, no friends) were unrelated. My mother . . . just scolded me, and said that my problems were due to a lack of effort on my part and that I should try harder. I grew up wondering how everybody else could somehow know the proper way to act. After all, I was much smarter than everybody in my class for things such as memory, math, pattern recognition, etc. I couldn't figure out how they would understand something like social interaction when I didn't get it despite being the smartest one. I just felt like some sort of freak with nobody else like me."[55]

Peter Hilts, Aspie, author, educator: "I am not satisfied to live in my own, isolated world. I want to be part of your world, especially the social universe. Unfortunately, I am an alien. I don't have the communications sophistication, emotional control or general intuition your society requires. I am a social incompetent—eager but awkward.

"We with Asperger's are intelligent enough to perceive our difference acutely. Our sense of abnormality is a persistent gloom . . ."[56]

aulrade: "How could anyone who's not an Aspie possibly understand how much it screws with your head and separates you from the world."[57]

aphonos (age 27): "You're so strange, people occasionally wonder if you're from another world.

"You don't try to be different, but you see most things from a very unique, very offbeat perspective. Brilliant to the point of genius, you definitely have some advanced intelligence going on.

"No matter what circles you travel in, you always feel like a stranger. And it's a feeling you've learned to like.

"Your greatest power: Your superhuman brain.

"Your greatest weakness: Your lack of empathy—you just don't get humans.

"You play well with: Zombies."[58]

Alyson Bradley: "Autism is like a web which is in the center and around it just some of the associated conditions people can have: PDD (Pervasive Developmental Disorder), OCD (Obsessive Compulsive Disorder), Social phobia, Anxiety, Bipolar, ADHD (Attention Deficit Hyperactivity Disorder), ADD (Attention Deficit Disorder), Dyslexia, Dyscalculia, Dyspraxia, Tourette Syndrome, speech disorders. It seems to depend on who you see, is what you get diagnosed with!"[59]

Colin White, a.k.a. CWhite978: "Throughout this absurd, pointless existence of mine, I have met time and again with people that act like I'm the one who needs to grow up and deal with my problem. I find this both amusing and aggravating. I have an exercise for NTs to help understand what it is like to be an Aspie: Go home, fill up a bathtub full of water, dunk your head underneath until you almost drown, come up for a breath, and then dunk again. Repeat for the rest of your life."[60]

Kathy Y Clark, a.k.a. Kat: "People are a total and absolute mystery to me. I am a people, but sometimes I don't feel like it. Sometimes I'd rather be anything other than a people.

"I'd rather be a dog or a tree or a scab on Julia Robert's elbow . . . anything but a person. I just find being a person is very difficult. Like what makes us a person? What makes us different from animals?

"Animals sniff each other's butts and go on about their business. Why can't we? They don't judge and dislike one another. They might fight, but over something important . . . like a chew toy. Mostly they just sniff and go."[61]

LF Morgen: "Ours is a self created world, where the individual on the autism spectrum can live without fear or confusion. It is conducting our own orchestra so that all the different aspects fit into a manageable tune . . . For people on the autism spectrum, life can be a labyrinth of stress, conflict, confusion and culture because, although born on this planet, its habits, customs and language are alien."[62]

On Eye Contact

Adrian, a.k.a. AS-4-L: "It's not just the lack of need to look someone in the eye . . . it just feels uncomfortable, I feel exposed and nasty. I don't know what's being asked of me. It's like the other person is trying to establish a bond that I'm not happy with, like a hug from a stranger."[63]

Griff: "If you watch NTs for a while, you will notice that they rarely actually gaze-lock. Their eye contact is friendly and gentle. You want to handle something like eye contact delicately as if it were something fragile and precious. You want to brush your gaze across another's as if with a fine paintbrush on a delicate canvas. You want to paint their eyes with yours as you would delicate eggs. As you move your eyes around envision paths being traced by them in the air and insure that the lines you make are pleasant ones. When you have completed this, a working of perhaps between one half of a second and a breath, you should be able to relax and make simple eye contact. Think of it as the docking of two spacecraft. It cannot be done well recklessly.

"The more difficult matter, however, is figuring out just what in the hell you're saying so you don't mistakenly say, 'I want you to take out your samurai sword, and shave my butt,' or 'I like children. I like your children.' It's a language all its own, part of it instinctive and part of it cultural. However, immediate gaze locking is almost always taken as a sign either of hostility or sexual advance.

"However, sometimes I do like to pick random women and give them my best 'psycho' gaze. Hehehehe, it's fun to watch them turn all white and cower away, HAHAHAHAHA! Carve RIGHT INTO the ray of their vision like a blunt sword, hehehe! They never see it coming![64]

Elizabeth Trosper, a.k.a. Spokane_Girl: "Luckily not many people forced me to look at them. I will look at people if I feel comfortable or if they have something interesting on them such as their fat or they are in a wheelchair or I like what they have on, or they have an ugly mole on their face, etc."[65]

Brains_&_Burgers: "I can't concentrate if I'm looking at someone—I won't hear/absorb what they are saying, or if I'm talking I'll lose any hope of concentrating or staying on track with what I'm talking about. I'll probably lose track anyways but I have a better chance if I'm not worrying about this eye-contact thing."[66]

Lofty: "I create the illusion of eye contact when necessary by staring between someone's eyes at their nose."[67]

On Empathy, Emotions, and "Mind Blindness"

Diamonddavej: "Up until a few years ago, I didn't realize people had emotions. It's not something I considered. It's not even something I knew I should consider—just like being blind to it."[68]

Shanti Perez, a.k.a. shantishanti: "I am always forthright, but often not sure what I'm feeling or how to sort out my feelings, so I am a what-you-see-is-what-you-get person. I live in the moment. My facial expressions do not even guarantee which emotion or state of mind I am in. So I probably send confusing signals to other people as well, which is counterproductive, isolating me from people when I really want people to be friendly toward me."[69]

BK_G: "I think the difficulty is that we cannot verbalize the emotions we are feeling. Because we cannot relate to the feelings others put words to, we cannot clearly identify what we are feeling, even to ourselves. It would be a bit like a colorblind person trying to communicate the color spectrum. With no vision of it in the first place, and no way to connect the verbal references to anything we experience, we are simply incapable of describing some feelings, despite feeling the same as what NTs might feel."[70]

fractalcurves: "I can't get into people's minds. I don't know what they want or what they feel unless I've been in the same situation in the past. I don't even understand my own feelings, let alone understand how other people feel. If you give me a scenario of something that hasn't happened to me before and ask me how I would feel in that situation, I will not be able to give you an answer."[71]

Sheila Schoonmaker: "I don't doubt it will appear to most people that AS people lack empathy, but that's only because NTs can't understand why they're getting the wrong impression about Aspies. Aspies need to be cognitively taught how to interpret the inconsistency between the feelings Aspies are aware of that others are experiencing (i.e., body language) versus what these others are orally saying. Understanding non-verbal messages comes intuitively easy for neurotypicals when the messages are coming from other NTs, because NTs share the same body signals while joining it with a different audible message. It's that illogical combination which throws Aspies into confusion."[72]

Katie (age 22): "There's a big difference between the clinical definition of empathy, and the common usage of the word.

The clinical definition of empathy is: 'KNOWING what someone else is thinking and feeling.' ... The common usage of empathy is 'Not being a jerk.'"[73]

b9: "With people in real life, I cannot imagine what they feel unless they say so in unambiguous terms, even if I look at them to see the expression on their face, I cannot tell, so I rarely bother to look."[74]

Liopleurodon (age 27): "I may come across as uncaring because I don't read the indications of what the other person is experiencing. I would care if I knew what was going on . . ."[75]

Danielismyname: "I don't have empathy —I have care, compassion and guilt however (much like most people with ASDs), all of which [feelings] are absent from Sociopaths, so those who equate ASDs to being a Sociopath are in error."[76]

tharn: "So what behavior is it that they expect in order for me to be labeled 'empathetic?' Do I have to be able to read the emotions people are hiding, or not fully expressing? Maybe they should learn how to express their emotions properly. I know any emotion I feel, I either express honestly or keep it to myself, and I don't expect others to read my mind—is that so much to ask of others?"[77]

Willard: "Lessee . . . Aspies spend their lives in a world that doesn't understand them or care to. We are treated as though we are worthless, lazy and weak because our brains are wired a little bit differently than average and we don't always respond the way normal, boring people do. Therefore, our feelings are stupid or just don't matter. And yet WE'RE the ones with no empathy?"[78]

On Employment

Adrian, a.k.a. AS-4-L: "So you can have AS *and* have what some might consider a successful life, but there is no guarantee of this at all. I was lucky in that I can make a career from my interest, but your special interest might be the cigars most loved by Winston Churchill, and if it is you're kinda screwed."[79]

userg: "I've been at the same company for 20 years and all of a sudden, out of the blue, they've decided to include in my performance review that I need to improve my 'social skills.'"[80]

April Anjard, a.k.a. liloleme (age 40): "I hate it when I'm in a job interview and they ask me 'are you a team player?'.... UHHHHHHHH"[81]

curiouslittleboy (age 20): [responding to **liloleme**] "Seriously though, what do they even MEAN by that anyways?"[82]

On New Situations and Change

Emma L.J. Walker, a.k.a. Belfast (age 35): "Surprises—in other words, alterations due to forces outside myself (from other people or the environment—physical, social, economic, etc.) are inherently unpleasant and destabilizing events, even when 'pleasant' in content.

"I can't snap my fingers & suddenly 'be ready' for whatever novelty I'm confronted with—it takes ages for me to 'settle in' & get comfortable with anything new."[83]

On Friends

nettiespaghetti: "I think that in general most people want to be accepted, even people with Asperger's. In my case part of me wants to have friends that understand me, but yet I don't like having people over at my house and I don't like making small talk, I don't like working with a lot of people or going to parties; I enjoy being by myself most of the time. But does simply the desire to want to have any friends at all mean that I don't have Aspergers? I don't think so. I would think that would lean more towards being anti-social. But then, I am no psychiatrist by any means. I just know that people with Aspergers do have friends often-times (from what I've read anyway), or at least one friend that they talk to, and they get married, etc. That requires friendship . . . ?"[84]

Evguenia Ignatova, a.k.a. fractalcurves: "Neurotypicals are less able to accept people with Asperger's because they cannot imagine what it's like to have a brain that works in a different way. Moreover, those with Asperger's are more gullible and it can sometimes be dangerous to give oneself in to a friendship with a neurotypical. Someone with Asperger's could theoretically be able to form a lasting friendship with someone who shares their disorder because of their similar ways of thinking and similar behavioral traits. However, there is one personality trait that could make this kind of friendship difficult to happen: the narrow nature of interests of people with Asperger's Syndrome. Given the relatively rare incidence of autistic disorders, about 6 or 7 in 1,000, it would be very difficult for someone who has the disorder to find another autistic person who shares the same interest. Relationships between two people on the autistic spectrum are usually interest-based since autistics tend not to do small talk. Therefore, in a friendship between two autistic people, one person would most likely have to adjust to the other in order for the friendship to function."[85]

jinxed: "It doesn't matter how hard I try, I can't keep friends. I think the time has come to say 'stuff it' and just be happy with my family. I've recently been chatting to a few people online, and I've recently had a misunderstanding or some sort of let down from all of them! I'm not a horrible or obnoxious person. Why do people dislike me so much?"[86]

dansa727: "I suffer from a moderate form of Aspergers. I also suffer from severe borderline personality and bipolar 1 disorder. Life's not easy for me, I work a decent job, but I get easily frustrated with my co-workers. I also lack social skills of any degree, and have no friends in life, my old friends have disowned [me] from high school."[87]

On Romance

JakeWilson: "On love, maybe we won't ever find a girl for us, but I just try to remember that I can't get any more single than I am right now."[88]

Adrian, a.k.a. AS-4-L: "Before my diagnosis I've always done my best, you know? I mean, God loves a trier. It usually takes me a while to get comfortable enough around someone to talk at least semi-freely instead of being all tight and nervous and self-conscious. It's bad enough with everyday people, but faced with a girl I find attractive . . . it seems to render me fairly useless.

"Now that I know what is wrong with me the fear of failing is stopping me [from] trying. I seem to resign myself to 'this isn't going to work so why bother' right from the outset."[89]

Joseph Sanchez, a.k.a. malithion2 (age 20): "I find with my AS I have to know a girl for a year before I start to feel comfortable around her."[90]

ToadOfSteel (age 20): "By the time I'm ready to begin something, I've been relegated to 'friend zone' due to lack of responding to any romantic overtures beforehand . . ."[91]

Keirts (age 30): "And I still can't read sexual and/or romantic signals from women. Not if my life depended on it, not until they walk up to me naked (happened once, she was rather frustrated; she could read my signals somehow but I couldn't read hers), and even then I was thinking 'Gee, she must be rather warm if she's taking her clothes off.'"[92]

On Being Alone

prillix (age 23): "If you are like me, yeah, being alone can feel great, compared to the alternative, rejection. After spending years and years of trying, oh so trying to fit in, sometimes it feels like nothing can be better than not trying, cause by not trying, there is no failure."[93]

Tohlagos (age 37): "Right now, I am content with being alone. Peace and quiet are nice and I move at my own pace.

"Other times, I do feel having some level of intimacy would be nice, but then I remember many things I would rather forget and revert back to being content of being alone."[94]

Eric "Pundit" Whalen: "Being alone is comfortable but having at least one good friend would be nice. Two or three if life is, as I am expecting, a scripted reality show."[95]

Aurore (age 18): "I do not want to be alone . . . I am definitely reaching for the life I feel I deserve, one with deep bonds in it. I feel a deep need to be with people. I'm fascinated by them; I just can't connect with them easily."[96]

Shanti Perez, a.k.a. shantishanti: "I give up and the ice forms around me and it grows so thick I become oblivious to those around me, focusing only on my interests. The humans in my life may feel rejected or invisible, too, but I don't know how to help this. Perhaps it is lucky, too, that I am writing this now, because in six months I may no longer be able to see what is happening. I may deny it and say others suffer inadequacies that are not my problem. I hope not but the way things are going I don't see myself staying connected to the people around me for much longer."[97]

aspiartist: "I think I've given up entirely on human beings. It isn't something I recommend though."[98]

hal9000: "I've always been a loner. I don't enjoy it but to me it's the lesser of two evils. Whenever I am forced to interact socially I get drained and I need the downtime by myself to recharge. Also most of the people I work with are liars, gossips and downright wicked. I just wasn't made for this life. I don't want to sound negative but it is just reality."[99]

Shawn Grannell, a.k.a. sgrannel: "Would I be better off married? Might raising parrots be better for me than raising children? I don't foresee becoming a hermit or an animal hoarder, though."[100]

On Anger Management

Aspies commonly experience high levels of frustration and anxiety as a product of their social inabilities, giving rise to anger. Characteristic lack of impulse control may also contribute to hostile outbursts, which further hamper the Aspie socially. Those who recognize their anger issues can benefit from therapeutic classes, or from the outspoken ideas expressed by their Aspie peers.

GroovyDruid: "Anger resides in your universe . . . As soon as you start to feel the anger . . . stop and become twice as angry . . . See, anger, fear, confusion and other unwanted emotions are only powerful in your internal universe as long as you can't control, manipulate, extend, contract, and generally run circles around them. But if you take your anger and order it to become twice as severe you actually take responsibility for the emotion. You are saying, 'I caused this emotion and I can cause some more if it pleases me. I am a god in my inner universe. Heh heh . . .' When you acknowledge you are a cause, then you stop being an effect—in this case, of your anger."[101]

Rick Hatfield, a.k.a. rixter: "Zen meditation is a highly effective way to learn to manage emotions, and also to manage the mind in general. You don't have to become Buddist, the basic meditation technique is actually used in all sorts of Christian and Islamic traditions, as well. All you do is sit quietly and observe yourself. Don't try to suppress your thoughts & emotions; just observe them without engaging them—like watching a movie. If anger arises, you simply note that you're feeling anger, & you let it go. You don't follow up on it & get caught up in some long chain of thought, you just watch. This eventually has the effect of giving you some extra perspective on your own thoughts & emotions . . . it's surprising how well this can work to diffuse a bad mood or obsessive thought. It teaches you to become calm and centered."[102]

A Look at Defiance

GM (age 19): "Christdamn!

She's at it again!

Now it's, 'I'm changing the computer passwords if you don't get a job by the end of June.'

Does she know NOTHING about Aspergers?

She claims to love me but she has no knowledge of our varied coping mechanisms, how we work, how difficult it is for us to find work in an environment which supports us . . . she knows nothing!

Does anyone have any suggestions on how I deal with her, sans snapping her neck and incinerating the body with oxidized elemental magnesium?

And when I try to argue back, she yells back about me threatening her or some-such crap and telling ME to stop yelling!

God . . . it feels good to get this off my chest.

She makes me want to take a baseball bat to her spine so she knows what it's like to be crippled. I'm socially crippled she'd be physically. Sounds fair.

And she has the f***ing gall to say she raised me! Stupid bitch, I raised myself. I could have made her life hell but I repressed nearly every trait I possessed.

If she had raised me worth a damn, I sure as hell wouldn't be in this position."[103]

On Depression and Suicide

Pat (age 21): "Are people with Asperger's more likely to commit suicide? From the time I was 13 or so until last year . . . I was extremely suicidal. There were times when I would go for months straight thinking of suicide and ACTUALLY planning on doing it. I don't know why, but for once in my life I haven't been suicidal. I can't find any kind of logical answer for why I am not suicidal, but there is a possibility that upon finding out that I have Asperger's and accepting it I no longer feel 'different.' I wonder if most people are relieved upon hearing that they have Asperger's?"[104]

866 (age 18): "Depression goes hand-in-hand with Asperger's and suicide goes hand-in-hand with depression. You do the math."[105]

Pat (age 21): "I think that the depression is caused from Aspies feeling 'different.' I don't know if I am wrong though, that was the case for me anyways."[106]

Shanti Perez, a.k.a. shantishanti: "I feel hopeless. I want to seal my lips together with E6000. I want a shutter in the middle of my office door—one that I can open when it is dinner time so that I can receive my plate and send it back when I am finished. I don't want to come out any more; it hurts too much.

"I don't know what to think or say anymore. I wonder when the ice will become too thick for me to connect. I feel it hardening now. I know it is not long. I am unable to change the way I think, the way I look, my unintended facial expressions, the way I try to systemize everything, even people, making them so that they are structures with predictable behaviors that I can analyze. But I still have feelings. I still feel pain."[107]

KatieRose212 (age 18): "I'm afraid that I AM suicidal. (You should look on my computer, I have been writing and planning how to kill myself for ages) and I swear if I have one more bad day I might just carry out one of the plans!!!

"But yeah . . . ever since finding out I had AS at age 13 has sent me into this spiraling depression that just won't go away. And I'm afraid that I am taking every day as it comes, and if life f***s me up, the only thing I can do is cut myself and cry myself to sleep hoping that it will all go away . . ."[108]

krex: "I was suicidal from 16-26 and still think of it as a possible solution to the life long dilemma of being on planet earth.

"I haven't abandoned suicide but figure I will try and learn as much as I can and can always kill myself in the future if I feel I just can't deal with the pain anymore. I try and keep my life balanced with the things that give me some pleasure (my interests) and keep my stressors down as much as possible."[109]

DanteRF (age 21): "The answer is really no. If someone that has AS, gets depression, then yes. Since AS itself has no bearing towards suicide I say no.

"I have depression and have tried, and failed of course."[110]

Jon West, a.k.a. Hodor (age 19): "Without looking at a piece of valid, unbiased data, it's impossible to say whether suicide is more common among people with Asperger's than among the general NT population. I suspect it is higher, not necessarily because there is a chemical link between AS and depression, but because a byproduct of AS is social isolation.

"Some people with AS can deal with social isolation. Great. But others can't, so that makes them depressed, question the reason for living, and ask themselves if there's any point in carrying on."[111]

Epitaphs

Postperson (age 52): "'You want me to do *what*?'"[112]

Danielismyname: "'Wings didn't work.'"[113]

Olivia Dvorak, a.k.a. poopylungstuffing (age 33): "Here lies little poopy dead . . . her brain was made of gingerbread . . . forget the rest of the poem . . ."[114]

oomogi (age 48): "When I die bury me deep, put two speakers by my feet, put some headphones on my head, and always play the Grateful Dead."[115]

normally_impaired (age 27): "He went through life and said aw-f**k it and wouldn'cha know he kicked the bucket."[116]

subliculous: "'I'll have four white castles and an onion ring, please."[117]

ApostropheX: "'Loved.' It is simple, worthy, and grammatically ambiguous."[118]

LOOKING FORWARD

*"And it must follow, as the night the day,
thou canst be false to any man."*

—Hamlet

Of the AS adults who have lived their lives without realizing their condition, some have been fortunate enough to find a career (or a career has found them) that suits their interests and keeps them effectively employed. Many are able to live independently, some marry successfully. Other AS persons struggle futilely with underemployment or unemployment and fall into desperation. Many have difficulty with the independent-living skills that require executive function. As a coping strategy, some self-medicate with drugs or alcohol. The terrain of Aspiedom is littered with broken relationships. Somersaulting difficulties for the Aspie; a waste of potential for all humanity.

Until we had a concept, a name, we couldn't do anything. We simply had no awareness, no category other than "weird," no window through which to view the behavior of an adult in Aspiedom. No one could take heed of AS persons or appreciate and nurture their strengths or support them in finding their way toward personal and social development. We did not have a clue.

For the three generations of (still living) adults who grew up knowing they were different, but having no name to put to that difference, no explanation or context for their communication/social difficulty, we can at last embrace the spectrum of autism. The formerly denied can now, once they are aware of and identify with Asperger's Syndrome, grasp their own "aha!" memories of growing up blind as to who they are.

As AS persons stated for themselves in the "Aspies Speak" chapter, they, almost universally, find great relief and satisfaction in becoming wise to the nature of their difference. And as no one lives in a social vacuum, aware families and acquaintances are at last able to assuage their angst and view their "different" dear ones in a revised context.

But after awareness comes adjustment. Neither personal acceptance nor acceptance by family and acquaintances is immediate; the course of adjustment to new insight is a process. Peter Hilts, Aspie author and educator in Colorado Springs, has developed a graphic to illustrate this process.[1]

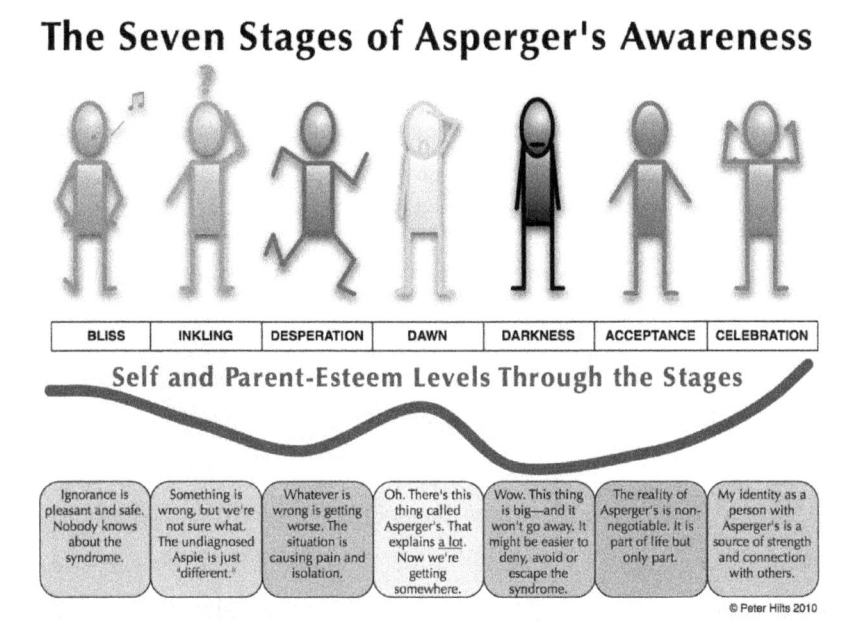

The Seven Stages of Asperger's Awareness

BLISS	INKLING	DESPERATION	DAWN	DARKNESS	ACCEPTANCE	CELEBRATION
Ignorance is pleasant and safe. Nobody knows about the syndrome.	Something is wrong, but we're not sure what. The undiagnosed Aspie is just "different."	Whatever is wrong is getting worse. The situation is causing pain and isolation.	Oh. There's this thing called Asperger's. That explains a lot. Now we're getting somewhere.	Wow. This thing is big—and it won't go away. It might be easier to deny, avoid or escape the syndrome.	The reality of Asperger's is non-negotiable. It is part of life but only part.	My identity as a person with Asperger's is a source of strength and connection with others.

Self and Parent-Esteem Levels Through the Stages

© Peter Hilts 2010

Each stage has its own characteristics, and each person moves through the stages at his own pace. Important to note: The last stage depicted here actually goes one step further than mere "acceptance."

Along with acceptance comes an energized, renewed concept of self—an anchor of identity when one in Aspiedom and those persons who care about him are ready for the "reset" button. Only then, with a finger depressing that button, does final stage become celebration!

Now, with our growing awareness of AS adults the challenge becomes how to proceed. A lot of questions are in front of us. How is an AS adult identified? By whom? Does he want a label? What would an AS label mean to a newly informed sense of self? How can individual ability and impairment be evaluated? How can vulnerability and naiveté be assessed? How can strengths be identified and satisfied? How should the self-aware AS person go about maximizing his renewed self? How can an awakening social structure incorporate or interface with the newly found heterogeneity? What trials must be passed as we embrace autistic diversity? What are our expectations? Do AS persons have to "fit" the NT model?

If "yes" is your answer to the last question, think again! Consider this exchange from *Star Trek, The Voyage Home*:

Gillian to (Aspie-like) **Spock:** "Are you sure you won't change your mind?"

Spock: "Is there something wrong with the one I have?"

During my correspondence with Asperger's Syndrome adults, as I got permission for quotes, I found that most Aspies, in their new awareness, do not want to change or do away with their Aspieness. They are not broken and they do not want to be fixed. They are whole, often very talented human beings with their characteristic abilities and "stamp of nature!" This idea, along with a hint for going forward, is well articulated in a recent email from AS person Denise Junk: "I feel like the Aspie neurology may hold some value to society as a whole. I think of us as a bit like an oil field before the invention of the combustible engine. If the right person could uncover our value and how to tap it . . . there lies a resource."

Hans Asperger himself recognized that although the symptoms and problems change over time, the overall condition is static. He wrote that "'in the course of development, certain features predominate or recede, so that the problems presented change considerably. Nevertheless, the essential aspects of the problem remain unchanged. In early childhood there are the difficulties in learning simple practical skills and in social adaptation. These difficulties arise out of the same disturbance which at school age cause learning and conduct problems, in adolescence job and performance problems and in adulthood social and marital conflicts.'"[2]

No doubt, trying to "fix" or suppress the Aspie, trying to manipulate him, trying to change him to fit the NT model, is not the social solution. It is not the personal solution. The effort itself could be counterproductive because the differences between NT persons and AS persons in sensory processing, communication and cognition are neurobiological in origin, and, therefore, mostly immutable.

However, awareness, appreciation, and integration are legitimate goals. What serves universally is that every adult, AS or NT, be able to explore his potential, to keep the mind that life gave him and to extract his personal oil field.

What's In A Name?

Up to now, the American Psychiatric Association has included the designation "Asperger's Syndrome" in *The Diagnostic and Statistical Manual of Mental Disorders*. Currently, however, the group is proposing to revise its definition of "Autism Spectrum Disorder" to subsume the reference to "Asperger's Syndrome." The proposed revised edition of the manual, to be available in May 2013, looks like this:

American Psychiatric Association, Copyright 2010
Autism Spectrum Disorder
Must meet criteria 1, 2, and 3:
1. Clinically significant, persistent deficits in social communication and interactions, as manifest by all of the following:
   a. Marked deficits in nonverbal and verbal communication used for social interaction
   b. Lack of social reciprocity
   c. Failure to develop and maintain peer relationships appropriate to developmental level
2. Restricted, repetitive patterns of behavior, interests, and activities, as manifested by at least *TWO* of the following:
   a. Stereotyped motor or verbal behaviors, or unusual sensory behaviors
   b. Excessive adherence to routines and ritualized patterns of behavior
   c. Restricted, fixated interests
3. Symptoms must be present in early childhood (but may not become fully manifest until social demands exceed limited capacities)[3]

Here is my take on the proposal: (1) Having a name is good; (2) Recognizing autism in that name is good; (3) Having a more specific qualifying name is good. (4) Having that qualifying name be the name of its discoverer, Hans Asperger, is very good; (5) Having that name be called a "disorder" is not good; 6) Having a diagnosis that, as proposed, appears to be written to assess only children, not adults, is not good; i.e., if an undiagnosed adult on the autistic spectrum does develop a peer relationship (see 1-c) and marries, can he, in his future, not be diagnosed an AS person? If he is diagnosed prior to marriage, then weds, is he then officially undiagnosed? (7) In conclusion, the revised nomenclature should be "Autism Spectrum/Asperger's." As we uncover subtypes, additional slashes could be added. That's the best.

Autism, including Asperger's Syndrome, is not limited to any particular nation; it is worldwide. As the above proposal is only for The American Psychiatric Association, its influence internationally and its impact on other diagnostic criteria cannot yet be determined.

In the historically ever-changing world of psychiatric diagnoses we are reminded that such designations are timely, committee drawn and not absolute. *And no matter what the nomenclature, it does not change the neurology.*

Regardless of the language or the diagnostic tool used to identify the condition, a label can be disarming, especially if announced to others. A brand does not take into account one's personal feelings, interests, or desires. The bearer of a diagnostic tag becomes secondary to that tag and may lose a sense of personal uniqueness. The stamp itself prefaces one's persona.

Conversely, by labeling, an AS person may gain an identity that makes sense to him, if previously he felt like a misfit. He may be able to access resources, create a plan of action to maximize his potential and participate in research, which, without a label, would be unavailable.

Because any label is important to the individual, it is critical that it be the correct one! To date, resources of qualified professionals to accurately assess adult AS persons may be difficult to find (remember, the diagnosis is subjective). Hopefully, with recognition that Asperger's

Syndrome is not just for children, more specialized expertise for assessing adults will evolve.

And we can't leave out the possibility that the AS adult might not want or feel the need for an "official" label. When one is an Aspie, he no doubt has all the personal insight required to self-identify, thereby satisfying his own psyche as to his acknowledged differences.

Regardless of whether one has a professionally confirmed label or whether he has put a name to his condition himself, it is always his choice as to when or with whom he wants to share his inclusion as an Asperger's Syndrome person.

Progress

As we go to press, public and private agencies, governments and individuals are stepping up to address the goals of awareness, appreciation, and integration of neurodiversity.

An outgrowth of heightened AS awareness is an increased demand for the services of NT professionals in the field. Beyond facilitating employment, social-development programs such as life-skills training, mentoring, interest development, education, and, if desired, behavioral-modification programs will become important integrative tools. And as more AS adults continue to identify themselves and more NT persons become aware of AS adults' social needs, more programs will emerge. Here is a sampling of programs designed to optimize the abilities of Aspies:

- *The Autism Society of America*, whose motto is, "Improving the lives of all affected by autism," represents an "example of how autistic self-advocates and parent advocates, despite possible underlying differences in perspective, can collaborate to assist autistics, parents, and others who work with them."[4]

- *The National Autistic Society* (United Kingdom) maintains an amalgam of services, including schools, housing programs, social support, employment support, education and training, telephone help lines, and assessment training for professionals.[5]

- *The University of Leicester* (United Kingdom) is "leading on a national study to calculate the number of British adults with autism" and researching their specific transition needs. This is the "first government strategy on adults with autism and Asperger's Syndrome."[6]

- *The Autism Diagnostic Research Centre* (United Kingdom) tests adults for autism and "aims to help individuals' quality of life as well as help their partners, families and colleagues understand the condition."[7]

- *The Welsh Assembly Government* launched the Autistic Spectrum Disorder Strategic Action Plan, "which included a commitment to establish a group to identify specific issues that adults face and take forward work to tackle them."[8]

- *Asperger Adults of Greater Washington* offers URL links to Asperger organizations around the world. Besides the United States and the United Kingdom, as listed above, the following countries have organizations addressing Asperger's Syndrome: Argentina, Australia, Belgium, Canada, Chile, China, Costa Rica, Denmark, Finland, France, Germany, Hong Kong, Ireland, Israel, Italy, Japan, Netherlands, New Zealand, Peru, Poland, Portugal, South Africa, Spain, Sri Lanka, Sweden, Switzerland, Turkey, and Uruguay.[9]

Employment

We can now rethink the old employment paradigm of the workplace needing only "people persons" and of teamwork being the primary job virtue. We can branch out and grow jobs that value solitary work, original thinking, and detail-oriented work that can accommodate meticulous, honest, dependable AS persons. Positions that are not interactively intensive but, rather, are ability embracing will help integrate the Aspie. Persons in Aspiedom, instead of being left dangling apart on their limb of the social tree, will, with improved acknowledgement and support, get a new grip and will find themselves employed where their talents and abilities can be enhanced, celebrated, and paid for.

Here is a sampling of current projects supporting awareness, appreciation and integration in employment:

- In Britain, the *Autism Act 2009* was passed "to address some of the social disparities" experienced by people on the autism spectrum. With the act, "disability employment advisors are going to be receiving autism training. This training is designed to improve the support system for jobseekers with autism-spectrum disorders so that they can navigate the job market more effectively."[10]

- An *article at the Web site, http://www. guardian.co.uk/* suggests ways to give autistic people access to work, including:

    "Think about your recruitment policy. 'Look at the emphasis you're placing on communication skills: does the role really need those skills?'
    "Be absolutely precise in the job description.
    "Adjust your evaluation process during an interview.

"Make reasonable adjustments if someone is over-sensitive to bright office lights, background chatter or prefers to work at home; do what you can."[11]

- *Aspiritech*, a nonprofit Chicago (USA) company, "recently launched a pilot program to train high-functioning autistics as testers for software development companies."[12]

- *Mission Possible* is a directory for Asperger's Syndrome in North America. Services offered include: "Job readiness assessment; identification of career options; identification of workplace challenges; vocational life skills training; job search and placement; job coaching; employer education/sensitization; and post employment support."[13]

- *Specialisterne* is a Danish company that employs adults on the autistic spectrum to test software and other systems. It is "a model of how to turn a highly skilled yet misunderstood and underexploited element of the population . . . into productive and integrated members of the workforce."[14]

- *FACT* (Focus on All-Child Therapies) is a nonprofit Los Angeles, USA-based program that "assists potential employers in matching the skill sets of adults with autism to various job descriptions which enables a good fit for the employer and employee."[15]

Techno Training

The ability to interpret facial expressions is not innate for Aspies. For them, learning the meaning of facial expressions must be practiced, largely by rote. But to a degree, it can be done, and learning the basic expressions of others can help the AS person with socialization—connecting to the feelings of others.

- Enter the *iSet,* a face-recognition program. This "interactive social emotional toolkit" is a "tablet with a camera on one side and a screen on the other, like an oversized cellphone." The device is aimed at another person's face until a video image "appears on the screen, along with identifying labels such as 'agreeing,' 'disagreeing,' 'concentrating,' and 'confused.'"[16]

- *Second Life* is a virtual world created by Dr. Sandra Chapman with the University of Texas at Dallas. It enables its users to interact with each other through avatars. "Users can explore, meet other 'residents,' socialize, participate in individual and group activities, and create and trade virtual property."[17]

Therapy, Mentoring, Advocating

- *Cognitive Behavioral Therapy* is used primarily to help the Aspie manage anger and anxiety. "The objectives of CBT typically are to identify irrational or maladaptive thoughts, assumptions and beliefs that are related to debilitating negative emotions and to identify how they are dysfunctional, inaccurate, or simply not helpful."[18] This is done in an effort to reject the distorted cognitions and to replace them with more realistic and self-helping alternatives.

- *The National Institute for People with Disabilities of New Jersey* has initiated a project for Asperger's adults. The program will focus on social skills and will explore vocational and educational options. "The major emphasis will be to enhance appropriate social and behavioral skills in order to make meaningful social connections, enhance employability and promote involvement in the community at large."[19]

- The Essex campus of the *Community College of Baltimore County* (Maryland, USA) has hired a special-education teacher to help college students "organize their time and assignments and improve the skills that are second nature to most, like how much space goes between two people in a conversation or how to make gentle eye contact."[20]

- *At Keene State College* (New Hampshire, USA), fellow students act as 'social navigators,' introducing their own friends to AS persons as a way to change their 'outsider' status. They help AS persons "make small talk, date and get consent at every level of romantic advancement."[20]

- *At Marshall University*, the West Virginia (USA) Autism Training Center operates a program in which "graduate students work daily with students with Asperger's, reviewing assignments, helping with time management and teaching classroom etiquette. They take the students on field trips . . . to let them practice social skills."[20]

- *Jeffrey Deutsch,* developer of *A SPLINT* (ASPies LInking with NTs) is a life coach and presenter in Washington, D.C. He trains "businesses and other organizations in accommodating those with autism and Asperger's Syndrome." In turn, he helps the latter to navigate a mainly neurotypical world. But the essential difference here is that first and foremost, Dr. Deutsch is an Aspie himself.[21]

Other Bright Ideas

- *The Illinois Premise Alert Program Act* enables voluntary enrollment in a database that will alert emergency responders to special needs that might complicate an emergency situation.[22]

- *Autism and Asperger's Passion Celebration Day* was conceived by Joel Goyette, the twenty-three-year-old twin brother of Dana, an AS person, so that Dana and others with specific interests could connect "with one another and to share their passions." Participants at Celebration Day each has a table dedicated to their unique passion (interest) and can talk about it with attendees.[23]

- *The San Francisco State University Special Education Program* studied the perspective of adults on the autism spectrum to learn their feelings and recommend social supports. Representative experiences included "a profound sense of isolation, difficulty initiating social interactions, challenges relating to communication, longing for greater intimacy, desire to contribute to one's community, and effort to develop greater social/self-awareness." The recommendations of the eighteen participants included activities based on shared interests, structured social activities, communication supports and self-initiated strategies for handling social anxiety.[24]

- *The Asperger Information Card* was developed by Mark Winter and Bart Vogelzang, members of the aspergerinfo.com online community. The card is available for PDF download for personal use. The text is here:

Asperger's Information Card

Front side

"Asperger's Syndrome (AS) is an Autism-related condition. People with AS can be of above-average intelligence but think differently, leaving them at a disadvantage in social situations. They need routine, and may become distressed when their routine is disrupted. Often having one or more heightened senses, they're more sensitive to changes from their normal environment, again causing reactions of distress. AS symptoms, which often include not making eye contact, and difficulty in making and reading facial expressions appropriately, can vary widely between individuals with AS. When interacting with someone with Asperger's, it is advisable to let them answer in their own words. More info at *www.aspergerinfo.com/knowmore* Emergency Contact: . . . ."

Back side

"Persons with AS, particularly when distressed, may not answer "yes/no" questions correctly. Please identify and remove the cause of their distress if possible, or guide them, with minimal physical contact, to a quiet place. Isolation often assists in recovery. *Raised voices, attempts to make eye contact, and threatening behavior will escalate their distress,* resulting in a range of possible reactions, including backing away, placing hands over the ears, breaking eye contact or involuntarily lashing out, either verbally or physically. POLICE OFFICERS AND SECURITY AGENTS: When dealing with a person with Asperger's Syndrome who is exhibiting signs of distress as detailed above, please use appropriate de-escalating strategies: lowered voice, non-threatening behaviors, minimal physical contact and isolation in a low stimulus environment."[25]

- Similarly, the *Autism Alert Card* is available in the United Kingdom. It is a "link-up" with the police force and the National Autistic Society and aims to "assist when police and those with an autism disorder or related conditions, like Asperger's Syndrome, come into contact." The card carries a help-line number for the NAS as well as personal details.[26]

Consider this: Some of the greatest advancements in the fields of art, science, music, math, and literature are the products of posthumously identified Aspies. Their unique ability for original perspective has resulted in contributions that have led the way across national boundaries, across cultural implications, across race, and across millenniums.

Neurological variability expressed as Aspie ability has propelled us through time and space (though the Aspie might tell you they are one in the same, *and* be able to tell you why). My guess is that the most important mechanical invention of all time was devised by an unnamed prehistoric Aspie who, in the fifth millennium BC, sat self-absorbed, perseverating about the process of transitory linear progression predicated on revolution of or around an axis. He gave us the wheel!

Indeed, the Asperger's Syndrome person is the one most likely "to . . . go where no man has gone before."[27] I, for one, look forward to what that means . . . .

VIEW FROM ASPIEDOM

Static Metaphor, Real-time Metaphor

"In my mind's eye."

—*Hamlet*

Magnifying Glass Metaphor

From the time I began studying, then writing about Asperger's Syndrome, I've been puzzling, trying to create an analogy or metaphor to explain just what the view from Aspiedom must look like. What kind of imagery might I use to convey the essence of the difference in the way an Aspie senses/processes stimuli as opposed to the sensing/processing experience of a neurotypical person (NT)? What quick mental picture would epitomize these disparate realities?

My first conceptualization was that of an Aspie with a face-sized magnifying glass permanently held to his field of vision. Through this, he is seeing some phenomenon up close and in exquisite detail. If he shifts focus, he sees one, then another point of interest, in a serial fashion. He can see only one intensely detailed point of interest at a time. It absorbs his attention. The Aspie may gain "encyclopedic knowledge" of a particular topic captured in that focus.

However, notice here that the area around the edges of the magnifying glass is *out of focus*. Light comes through this peripheral circumference, but no clear images can be discerned. They are but a blur. And this is the *context* for what the Aspie is viewing *in* focus! But he has no way to clearly assess the connection between what is in his focus and the milieu surrounding it. His focused pictures are a part of a more comprehensive *what*? Fitting the details into the whole is a struggle that is confusing and exhausting. When one cannot make contextual "sense" of his input or stimuli, one may opt to disregard all the extraneous images and cling to his private world of interesting minutiae. Or he will be awkward or frustrated in the continual effort to *make* the pieces fit into a model that he cannot fully grasp. So the magnifying glass becomes a metaphor for observed particulars of environmental interaction and of unrecognized context.

No Satisfaction: Real-Time Aspie Metaphor

Once I was comfortable with the magnifying glass image as a metaphoric illustration of the obscured Aspie view of the socio-emotional world about him, I found myself in the middle of what I came to realize was a simulated (inadvertently or purposefully) two-hour, real-time Aspie metaphoric experience!

In June 2008, my husband and I had just watched *Shine A Light*, a film by Academy Award-winning filmmaker Martin Scorsese that documented a Rolling Stones concert at Beacon Theater in New York City.

After leaving the IMAX theater, I had a sense of mental exhaustion that I deemed could only have been the result of watching this Rolling Stones concert! But how can a concert film be draining?

One would certainly assume that a film of a rock concert would look and sound much like the live concert. One might feel like he was in the audience or even perceive that he had an edge over the live experience by being shown some close ups and varying camera angles that the live audience might not get. He would be able to see all the performers, singing and playing their instruments together. He would see the stage design and witness all the action. He would almost be one of the fans pulsating in unison to the performance in a context defined by the embrace of the venue. He would have everything he needed to realize an experience greater than the sum of its individual parts. He could delight in the gestalt of synchronicity. It would all make such satisfying sense.

Oh, no. It didn't work that way. Our filmmaker gave us something different; he instead gave us his art. We were limited to viewing this "concert" through Scorsese's alternative *interpretation* of the live concert. The director's tools of cameras and gels allowed him to manipulate the footage to make his own counter-concert statement.

And what a statement Mr. Scorsese made. He cinematically chose to let us view *only the parts* of the performance. Literally, *parts*. We heard all the songs, all the words to the songs, all the music, but we got to *see* only parts. He showed us prancing legs, swaying backs, individual instruments, contorted faces, faces of duos, trios, guests, and band members, all playing what they play and singing as they sing. We saw the close-ups and the extreme close-ups, this angle and that angle. We did not want for detail, all in a thousand small "takes." He had the gall to *never* let us see the *whole* concert as it was happening!

So we got oddments and snippets. All the explicit particulars that one could not see as a live audience member, we saw. But now, we had no contextual place to put them! No basket of *meaning*. No way for us to relate these small takes to the total concert experience. This film was an entertaining tinkering with bitty bits.

Mr. Scorsese's *processing* of the event was indeed disparate from an actual concert experience. And it is this film's focus on bits and pieces indeed that brings us to the brink of Aspiedom. Now, just like an Aspie, with all those conjured close-ups, I could see and obsess over the smallest fascinating detail. That single four-inch thread from Keith Richard's raggedy headband dangling alongside his cheek monopolized my attention. And I could study the marvelous texture and shadowing of every fascinating crag in Mick's and Keith's faces. I could scrutinize the pockmarks in Keith's arm like craters on the moon seen through the finest telescope. The images were present, in your face and compelling, but what were they all doing here? What was the *meaning* of all these elaborate details? Where did they fit? What relevance did they bear?

Fragments alone do *not* add up to the satisfying experience of a live concert. Because we never got to enjoy the wide angle, the whole band relating to one another, on a stage, in an arena, with screaming fans, we never got to see the essence, the *context* for the details being presented. In this cinematic rendition, the defining boundaries of the event itself blurred into the ether.

So how could these plenary pieces amount to exhaustion? What generated the fatigue I felt, even though I enjoyed the thousand up-close points of view?

It was the mental gymnastics required to find relevance that taxed my viewing. In the effort to make the fragments *mean* something, I had to visualize the "takes" into my existing, experience-based model of what a concert is.

If I could not have placed these parts into that whole, my experience simply would have been a string of wonderful textured "take" beads strung around a phantom neck.

And I say this as one who does have a concert model in her head. Just think how difficult the extension of that effort to find meaning would be for one who had no whole concert model in his head!

How like the day-to-day social interaction for one in Aspiedom! The AS person hears words and sentences, sees people, and appreciates all the superabundant details. He zooms in on all the "parts" with acute clarity. But he struggles in social encounters to envelop those pieces into a social/emotional model to give them consequent meaning. And if he is exhausted after trying to fit into any social situation and needs time alone to zoom out for recovery, I now see why.

POSTSCRIPT

"Though this be madness yet there is method in 't."

—*Hamlet*

POSTSCRIPT is a collection of comments and conversations between Dylan and myself that took place as I researched and wrote *WWDYM*. As such, they did not become part of the text but rather have their own identity as garnishes.

April 2008

Regarding permission to write about him: I called to ask Dylan if he minded that I was writing a book about discovering his presence in Aspiedom. His answer: "Do *you* mind if I don't read it?"

May 2008

Regarding the "50¢ egg": On Mother's Day, Dylan called. I gave him just this one-paragraph example of what I had written in the **DYLAN "Aha!"** chapter. His comment: "I must have been a slow learner . . . Only one zero?!"

Regarding Aspie idiomatic language comprehension: I decided to test (on Dylan) the theory that Aspies do not "get" idiomatic language.

My husband and a friend were the first control subjects. The question was, what does the expression "when pigs fly" mean? Both persons responded that the expression means that "it will not happen," or "is very unlikely to happen." Two points for the NTs. Now for the Aspie, Dylan . . . I totally expected that as an Aspie he would take the literal route and would reply, "What do you mean? Pigs don't fly."

Phone conversation: Dylan is at work but picks up his phone. The usual greetings, then my question, "What does the expression 'when pigs fly' mean?" Without any hesitation, Dylan's response was, "Is that like when hell freezes over?" My theory disproved in a big way, at least on this occasion. Not only did he respond correctly to the idiomatic question, he took it to the next level; he nailed it with another idiomatic expression! Sweet! On hearing my delighted response, he said, using a simile, "I feel like I just won a contest!" Caveat: both the question and answer metaphors were traditional and well used linguistically. Dylan's response may have been different if the metaphoric question was original instead of one Dylan had probably already heard and had learned. (see also chapter **ASPIES SPEAK**)

"**Idiots.**" Phone conversation: While writing the chapter **DYLAN "Aha!"** knowing his continued propensity for anger directed at others, I asked him just what it is about others that makes him mad. He replied, "When they are idiots." Subsequently, I asked him in another phone conversation to make a David Letterman-style top ten list of the idiotic actions of others, thinking that it might make an enlightening addition here for NTs to understand what goes on in the Aspie mind. He responded that he couldn't do that; his list would be a whole book . . . .

June 2008

Regarding questions I had to accurately portray timing and sequencing of events: I phoned Dylan to ask how long his marriage to Aimee lasted. "Technically, a year and a half. Actually, about three weeks."

I also asked him what happened to his truck. (Why he doesn't have it anymore.) Note the very linear response: "The transmission went out. Then someone slashed the tires. Then the windows were broken. Then the city ticketed it, saying they were going to tow it. Then they towed it. . . ."

Standing corrected: Per another phone conversation to get the facts on the rugby collarbone issue, Dylan told me that he knew he was "dangerously insensitive to pain." I repeated back, "You know you are insensitive to pain?" **Correcting** me, he says, "No, I said I'm *dangerously* insensitive to pain."

November 2008

I had read time and time again about how often AS children are teased and bullied in grade school. Even though I had never heard of Dylan being teased, and frankly, knowing his aggressiveness, doubted that he was, I had to ask, just to be sure. I texted him the question, "Were you ever teased in school?" His prompt text message back was, "Are you high?"

February 2009

Speaking by phone with Dylan on his thirty-eighth birthday: Dylan: "I have a friend who has Asperger's worse than I do. What a dork!" Then, acknowledging his own apparent debility with relationships, says, "You know he's got it bad if he's asking *me* about girls!"

August 2009

I texted Dylan to ask if he would write a poem about what his life is like now, with Asperger's awareness. His same-day response, by text message:

> "Rough draft:
> It'll soon be apparent that I am no bard
> But actually TALKING to you fools is fucking hard
> Now thanks to this dude named Asperger
> We have a fancy euphemism for
> My previous label of social goddamn retard!"

November 2009

After reading the Introduction to *WWDYM*, where I wrote, "He has neither role modeled his way to a career . . . ," Dylan wrote on my page next to "role modeled," "What does that mean?"

December 2009
After Dylan read the DYLAN, "Aha!" chapter,
- Dylan reminded me that in the time period after Jason died, and before I got a grip on healing, "You cried all the time."
- I wrote that an autistic child may not know what's going on when another child cries. He wrote, "But we know how annoying it is."
- I wrote that an autistic child may take action just to see what happens. He wrote, "Ha! Should have seen me in my chem & physics labs in high school. Or on dates . . ."
- I wrote that Dylan begins work late to accommodate his need to sleep late. He wrote that "I don't sleep anymore."

- I wrote about AS persons' attention to detail. He wrote that "people were impressed when [as a small child] I saw the little insects on a poster depicting wild flowers."
- I included Jason's letter regarding Dylan's aggressive behavior. He wrote, "Doesn't anyone think it's strange that an 8th grader would write his own police report?"
- I wrote that Dylan's grades dropped slightly in eleventh grade. He wrote that he discovered "beer and girls."

Miscellaneous Aspie moments

Remembering back to the day fifteen-year-old Dylan drove a car: With the appropriate learner's permit in hand and me, the licensed driver, in the car, Dylan sat in the driver's seat as I began to instruct him on the use of the standard transmission. He turned on the key and with amazing know-how could drive using the required clutching and shifting of gears, *without my instruction.* Remembering back to my own experience of learning to drive, it was not easy and took practice. But Dylan amazed me so much at his inherent ability to just get in and drive, that I asked him how he learned so quickly. He said, "I watched . . . ."

A few years ago, Dylan was dating a woman from Brazil. He was on his way to Sao Paulo with her. I referred to the young lady as his "girlfriend." Dylan corrected me, saying he "did not know if she was his girlfriend or not!"

Last year, after hearing that many AS persons do not like being hugged, as in greeting, etc., I asked Dylan how he felt about hugging. He replied that it did not bother him, but he "did not know when to do it."

WRITTEN ILLUSTRATIONS/AWARDS/NOTES

The following awards were given to Dylan during his middle-school years.

The writings are from eighth-grade English class. In the assignment, i.e., "My idea of a perfect day is . . . ," the teacher wrote the topic sentence, or "prompt" on the chalkboard. The students' responsibility was to write a half page completing the prompt. Students were given credit if they completed the assignment, but the responses were neither read by the teacher nor graded as to content.

In his senior year in high school Dylan received the Bank of America award for excellence in Physical Science. He graduated with a lifetime membership in the California Scholarship Federation for "high standards in academic scholarship. . . ."

Dylan's awards shown here are juxtaposed with Dylan's writings to illustrate further the emotional/social status of an Asperger's Syndrome youth.

Award for outstanding scholastic achievement

MY FAVORITE TOY I HAD AS A CHILD WAS MY BARBIE-DOLL SIZED G.I. JOE FIGURE. I OWNED ALL KINDS OF ACCESSORIES TO PLAY WITH WITH MY G.I. JOE FIGURE, SUCH AS: GREEN MILITARY CLOTHES, CANTEENS, HELICOPTERS, GUNS, ETC. THE G.I. JOE FIGURE ALSO HAD A FUZZY HEAD TO LOOK LIKE HAIR. MY BROTHERS AND I USED TO BURN AND SHAVE SOME OF THE "HAIR" OFF TO MAKE STRANGE HAIRSTYLES, SUCH AS MOHAWKS. I ALSO TOOK A WOOD-BURNING PEN AND BURNED IN HIM TO LOOK LIKE BULLET WOUNDS. AFTER MANY YEARS OF FUN AND ABUSE, HIS LEGS AND ARMS BEGAN TO FALL OFF, SO I TOOK HIM OUT TO OUR BACK YARD, AND CREMATED HIM WITH LIGHTER FLUID.

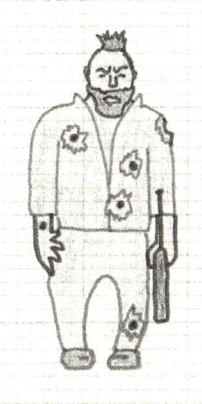

"My favorite toy"

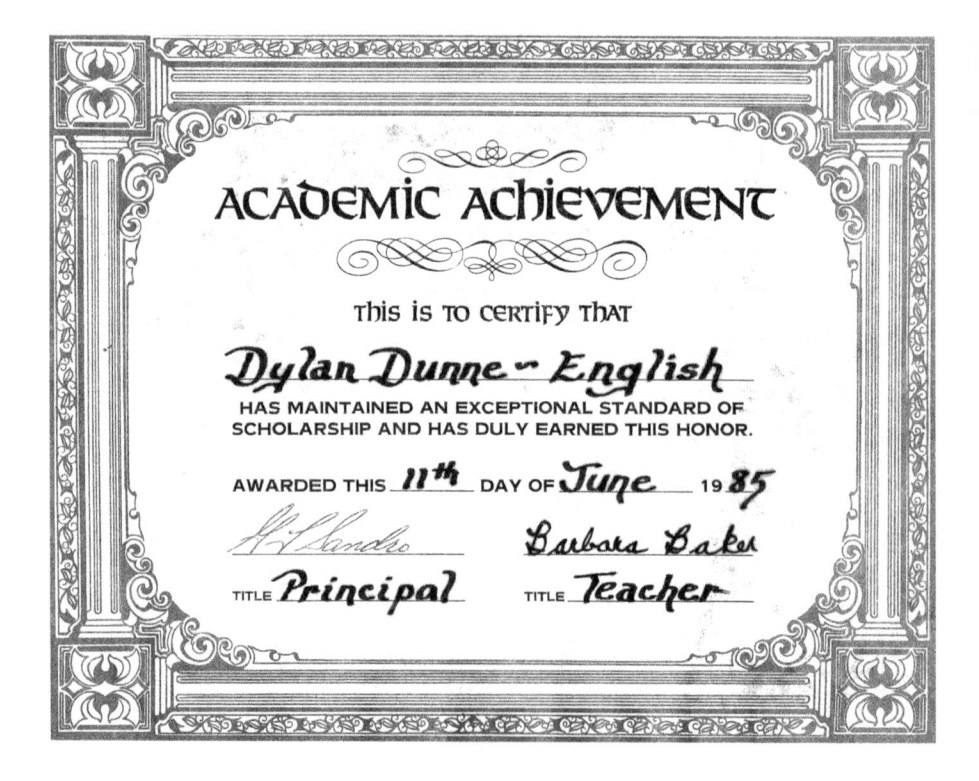

Award for exceptional scholarship in English

MY DESCRIPTION OF A PERFECT DAY: WHILE I'M WALKING TO THE BUS STOP ON A SUNNY, SPRING MORNING, I STUMBLE UPON A LAW 80 ROCKET LAUNCHER. SURPRISINGLY, I MANAGE TO SMUGGLE IT ONTO THE BUS. AS OUR BUS IS PULLING INTO THE SCHOOL'S DRIVEWAY, CECIL, OUR BUS DRIVER, DIES OF A HEART ATTACK. THE BUS RUNS INTO MR. PECCANTI AND CRASES, KILLING EVERYONE EXCEPT MIKE SKOLFIELD AND MYSELF. I THEN REMOVE MY ROCKET LAUNCHER FROM MY DUFFEL BAG, AND THEN, FIRING FROM MY SHOULDER, I APPLY THREE PROJECTILES TO THE SCHOOL AND ANOTHER TO THE OFFICE, BLOWING THEM INTO DEEP SPACE (ALONG WITH THE REMAINS OF THE TEACHERS). MIRACULOUSLY, ALL OF MY FRIENDS LIVE, AND ALL OF MY ENEMIES DIE. WOW! THEY REST OF THE DAY MY FRIENDS AND I CELEBRATE AT THE BOAT WORKS (AND GO SWIMMING AT FLOYD'S HOUSE AT NIGHT).

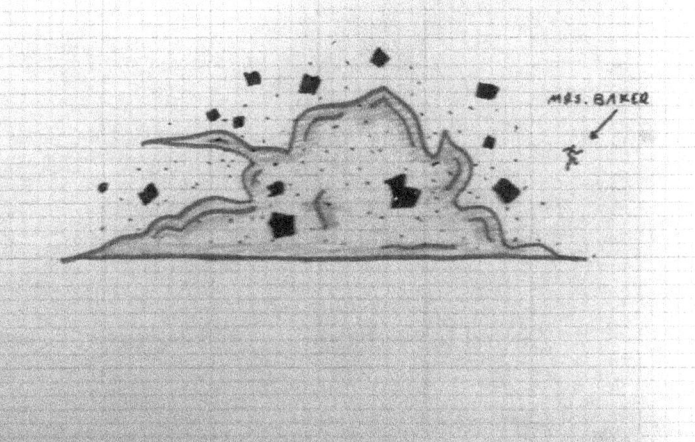

"A perfect day"

Award for outstanding achievement in math

THE CHARACTER FROM A MOVIE I'VE SEEN WHOM I WOULD MOST LIKE TO MEET AND TALK TO IS, SARGEANT KEVIN SHAWN, THE LEADING SENTRY CADET AT BUNKER HILL MILITARY ACADEMY, IN THE MOVIE <u>TAPS</u>. I WOULD LIKE TO MEET THE CHARACTER PLAYED BY TOM CRUISE BECAUSE I LIKE HIS MEANNESS AND CRAZINESS, AND WISH I WERE MORE LIKE HIM. IF I WERE ACTUALLY LUCKY ENOUGH TO MEET HIM I WOULDN'T REALLY KNOW WHAT TO SAY, SO I'D JUST ASK HIM SOMETHING LIKE," WHY'D YOU GO SO CRAZY WHEN EVERYONE WAS FALLING IN, AND NOT BEFORE? LIKE AT NIGHT?"

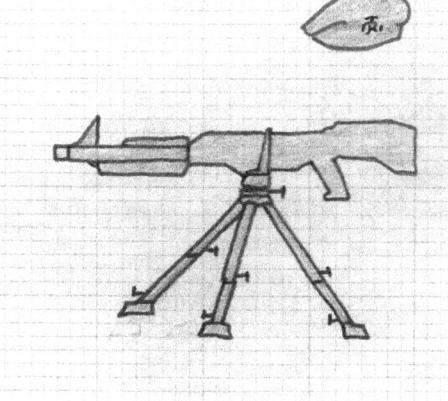

"Movie character I'd most like to meet"

Award for being a promising author

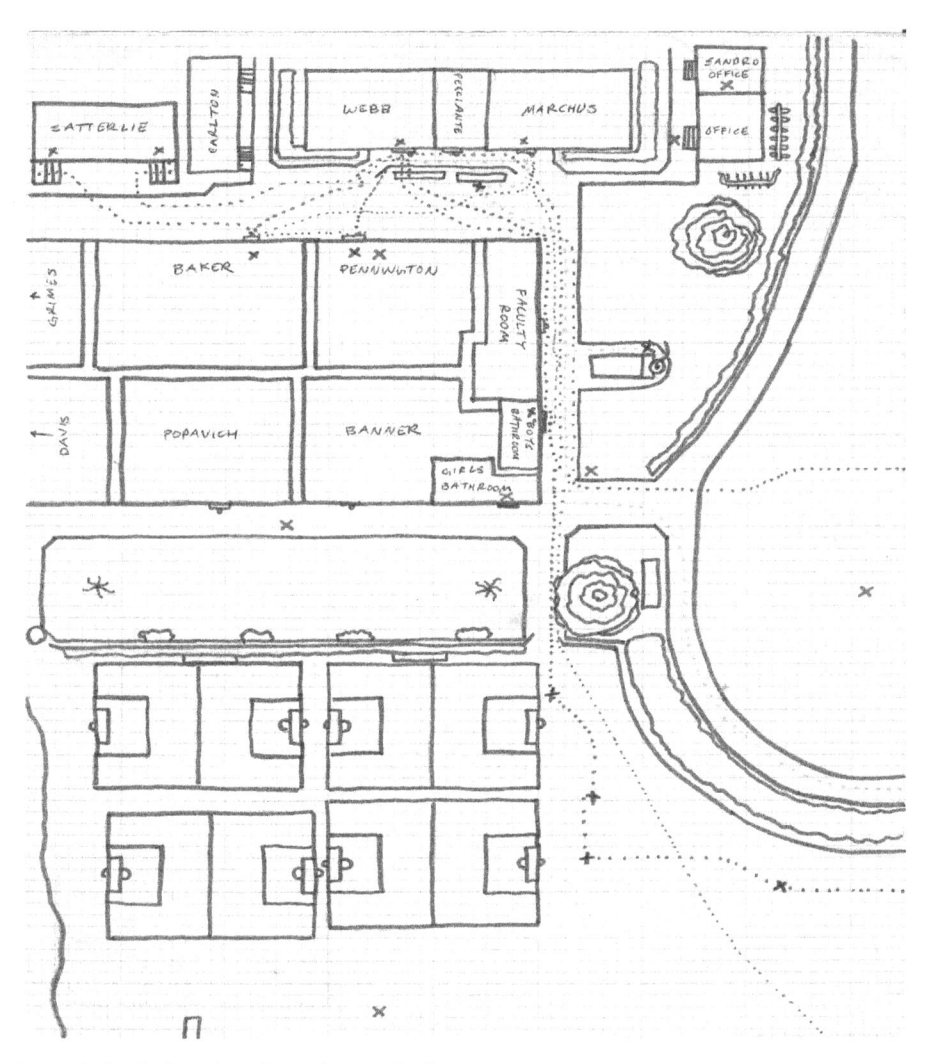

The original drawing is color coded to show footsteps taken at the various times of day. The darker Xs show places to avoid. The lighter Xs show places to stop. As this book goes to press, Dylan does not remember the significance of the drawing, but says that it's "disturbing." He also says he "does not remember why he was so bored (and why the girls' bathroom was one of my places to stop). Who knows, maybe a reader will offer a theory . . . ."

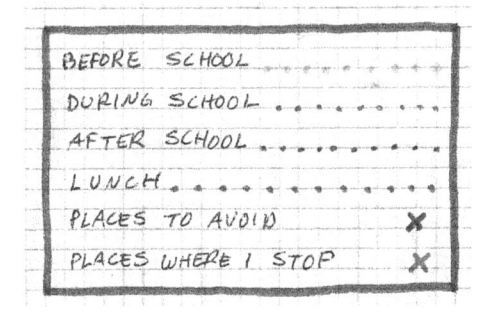

Campus conundrum

IF I COULD CHANGE ONE THING ABOUT MYSELF, IT WOULD HAVE TO BE MY TEMPER. THIS WOULD BE A HARD DECISION, SINCE I AM A VERY IMPERFECT PERSON, BUT I'LL SOON START TO LOSE FRIENDS IF I ALWAYS ARGUE AND FIGHT WITH THEM. MY TEMPER IS SO BAD THAT I OFTEN GET MAD AND HIT PEOPLE (EVEN GIRLS) OVER STUPID LITTLE THINGS. CHANGING MY TEMPER, HOWEVER, DOES NOT HAVE TO BE WISH, AND I PLAN ON DOING SO RIGHT AWAY.

"If I could change one thing"

BIBLIOGRAPHY

DYLAN
"Aha!"

1. Translation of "What Is Asperger's Syndrome?" August 2002 by the Tokyo Chapter of Autism Society Japan. http://www.autism.jp/asp_eng.html.

2. Public Autism Awareness, "Asperger's Syndrome," Copyright Paains 2001-2004. http://www.paains.org.uk/related/aspergers.htm.

3. Yahoo! Answers, 1/5/2008. http://answers.yahoo.com/question/index?qid=20080105114220AAQoUAf.

4. Life with Aspergers: "Aspergers and Sleep Disorders," posted by Gavin Bollard, 8/6/2009. http://life-with-aspergers.blogspot.com/2008/08/aspergers-and-sleep-disorders.html.

5. "All about Dylan," by Dylan Dunne, 1979.

6. Laboratoire de Neurosciences cognitives des troubles envahisssants du developpement, "Atypical sleep architecture and the autism phenotype," by Limoges E., Mottron, L., Bolduc C, Berthiaume C,

Godbout R, 2/2005. http://www.lnc-autisme.umontreal.ca/n45/index.php?option=com_content&view=article&id=109&Itemid=179.

7. HealthDay, "Asperger Syndrome Tied to Low Cortisol Levels," 4/2/2009. http://health.discovery.com/news/healthscout/article.html?article=625706&category=28&year=2009.

8. About.com: Autism, "Mood Disorders and Asperger Syndrome," by Lisa Jo Rudy, 7/6/2008. http://autism.about.com/od/aspergerssyndrome/a/moodsasperger.htm.

9. TCPalm.com, "Schools like Morningside Elementary walk fine line on where to place autistic students," by Colleen Wixon, 6/1/2008. http://www.tcpalm.com/news/2008/jun/01/30gtschools-walk-fine-line-of-where-to-place/.

10. revolutionhealth, "Biting and Autism," by Elizabeth Verdick, 4/8/2008. http://www.revolutionhealth.com/blogs/resilientmom/biting-and-autism-12819.

11. CBS11TV.com, "UTD Docs Use Online World To Treat Form Of Autism," by Ginger Allen, 7/9/2008. http://cbs11tv.com/health/aspergers.syndrome.treatment.2.767511.html.

12. NRC HANDELSBLAD, "Autism's double punishment," by Dick Swaab, 1/9/2009. http://weblogs.nrc.nl/swaab/2009/01/09/autisms-double-punishment-3/.

13. "All about Dylan," by Dylan Dunne, 1979.

14. O.A.S.I.S., Stephen Bauer, M.D., MPH "Asperger Syndrome," http://www.udel.edu/bkirby/asperger/as_thru_years.html.

15. Grandparents Raising Grandchildren, TM Trust NZ "How to cope with violent outbursts from a child with Aspergers," 11/2008. http://www.raisinggrandchildren.org.nz/webapps/site/75791/130050/news/news-more.html?newsid=211966.

16. AllExperts: Autism, "Asperger's and suspension from school," by Julia Erdelyi, 9/27/2006. http://en.allexperts.com/q/Autism-1010/Asperger-suspension-school.htm.

17. Autistic Spectrum Disorders Fact Sheet, "Humor and Conflict," by Marc Segar. http://www.autism-help.org/aspergers-guide-humor.htm.

DYLAN
"Ahhh!"

1. Personal email from Jim Sinclair, autistic adult and Coordinator, Autism Network International 7/15/07. www.ani.ac.

WHAT IS IT?

1. MSNBC, "Mild autism has 'selective advantages,'" by Sue Herera, 2/25/2005. http://www.msnbc.msn.com/id/7030731/.

2. The Westmount examiner, "Autism and Asperger's: The Mysterious Syndromes," by Marylin Smith Carsley, 1/21/2008. http://www.westmountexaminer.com/article-176414-Autism-and-Aspergers-The-Mysterious-Syndromes.html.

3. BBC News Online Magazine, "What Asperger's syndrome has done for us," by Megan Lane, 6/2/2004. http://news.bbc.co.uk/2/hi/uk_news/magazine/3766697.stm.

4. "Asperger Syndrome," Stephen Bauer, M.D., M.P.H., 1996. http://www.udel.edu/bkirby/asperger/as_thru_years.html.

5. "Asperger's Syndrome and Bipolar Affective Disease," Journal of Autism and Developmental Disorders, Vol. 18, No. 4, 1988. http://www.springerlink.com/content/k245p8uwt58707m7/.

CAUSES/EFFECTS/WHAT'S GOING ON

1. guardian.co.uk, "Disorder linked to high levels of testosterone in womb," by Sarah Boseley, 1/12/2009. http://www.guardian.co.uk/lifeandstyle/2009/jan/12/autism-prenatal-testosterone-womb.

2. azcentral.com, "Potential breakthroughs in Autism research," by Joe Dana, 5/28/2009. www.azcentral.com/12news/news/articles/2009/05/28/20090528autismresearch05282009-CR.html.

3. Sacramento Bee, "Study explores autism link to immune system," By Carrie Peyton Dahlberg, 1/25/2008. [pay to play archive] www.sacbee.com/health/story/661144.html.

4. suite101.com, "Autism and Immunity," by Stephen Allen Christensen, 10/18/2008. http://autism.suite101.com/article.cfm/autism_and_immunity.

5. Parents of Allergic Children—Virginia, "Pervasive Developmental Disorders (PDD) and Autism," 'The Structural Connection' www.

parentsofallergicchildren.org/autism_spectrum.htm (reprinted with permission from the Optometric Extension Program Foundation) http://www.oepf.org/.

6. blogspot sourced from BBC News online, Associated Press, MedPage Today, The Times, The Independent, "Fathers over 40 much more likely to have autistic children," 5/9/2006. http://autism-prevention.blogspot.com/2008/03/fathers-over-40-much-more-likely-to.html.

7. UC Newsroom, "Link confirmed between advanced mother's age, autism," Contact: Phyllis Brown, 2/8/2010. http://www.universityofcalifornia.edu/news/article/22790.

8. Suite101, "Theories on What Causes Autism," 'Rainfall Rates,' by Melissa Hincha-Ownby, 11/6/2008. Sourced from ScienceDaily Online, accessed 11/6/2008. http://autism.suite101.com/article.cfm/theories_on_what_causes_autism.

9. OneNewsNow, "Aborted baby DNA—'environmental factor' in autism," Charlie Butts, 5/5/2010. http://www.onenewsnow.com/Culture/Default.aspx?id=998666.

10. CAT.INIS, "Cortical folding abnormalities in autism revealed by surface-based morphometry," Society for Neuroscience, Wu Nordahl, et. al, 2007. http://cat.inist.fr/?aModele=afficheN&cpsidt=19210114.

11. "Intelligence, Asperger's Syndrome, and Learning Disabilities at MIT, 'Autistic Males Have Fewer Neurons in Amygdala,' Scientific American, 7/19/2006. http://bgrh.websitetoolbox.com/post?id=1270535.

12. Reuters, "Study maps brain abnormalities in autistic children," by Susan Kelly, 11/28,2007. www.reuters.com/article/idUSN2754212320071128.

13. e! Science News, "Faulty brain connections may be responsible for social impairments in autism," 6/12/2008. http://esciencenews.com/articles/2008/06/12/faulty.brain.connections.may.be.responsible.social.impairments.autism.

14. PubMed, "Differential fear conditioning in Asperger's Syndrome: implications for an amygdala theory of autism,", by Gaigg SB, Bowler DM, Dept. of Psychology, City Univ., London, Uk, 5/15/2007. http://www.ncbi.nim.nih.gov/pubmed/17321555.

15. BBC News, "Protein mutations link to autism," 6//21/2007. http://news.bbc.co.uk/2/hi/health/6221064.stm.

16. Science Daily, "Brain Imaging May Help Diagnose Autism," 1/10/2010. http://www.sciencedaily.com/releases/2010/01/100108101421.htm.

17. Aspies for Freedom, "Genetics Study links Autism to timing mechanisms," posted by Gareth, 3/7/2007. http://www.aspiesforfreedom.com.

18. Psychology Today, "The Imprinted Brain," by Christopher Badcock, Ph.D., 2/25/2010.
http://www.psychologytoday.com/blog/the-imprinted-brain/201002/lingering-lyonization-does-explain-the-genetics-aspergers-syndrome.

19. New York Magazine, 5/25/2008. "The Autism Rights Movement," by Andrew Solomon, http://nymag.com/news/features/47225/.

20. Huliq News, "Genes Associated With Asperger Syndrome, Empathy Identified," 7/15/2009. http://www.huliq.com/11/83570/genes-associated-asperger-syndrome-empathy-identified.

21. Science News, "Outside looking in: researchers open new windows on Asperger syndrome and related disorders," by Bruce Bower, 8/12/2006. http://findarticles.com/p/articles/mi_m1200/is_7_170/ai_n16690545/pg_3/?tag=content;col1.

22. Mail Online, "Rogue gene which can raise the risk of autism is pinpointed by scientists," by Fiona MacRae, 1/10/2008. http://www.dailymail.co.uk/health/article-507338/Rogue-gene-raise-risk-autism-pinpointed-scientists.html.

23. AMHC, "Gene Variant Allies Autism, Gastrointestinal Woes," by Amanda Gardner, 3/2/2009. http:www.amhc.org/poc/view_doc.php?type=news&id=117142&cn=20.

24. Reuters Health, from MSMBC web site, "Gene hSERT mutation and Asperger's Syndrome," 10/23/03. http://www.nvo.com/hypoism/clinicallyimportantneurotransmitterdeficiencies/.

25. canada.com, "A medical Pandora's box," Calgary Herald, 1/13/2008. http://www.canada.com/calgaryherald/news/theeditorialpage/story.html?id=f44c994a-54d1-4e1c-b772-42b8e4e491a9.

26. The Nation, 7/11/2010. http://www.nation.com.pk/pakistan-news-newspaper-daily-english-online/Regional/14-Jul-2008/Gene-research-heightens-hope-for-curing-autism.

27. Parents of Allergic Children, "From Attention Deficit Disorder to Autism: A Continuum," by Patricia S. Lemer M.Ed, 1996. http://www.parentsofallergicchildren.org/autism_spectrum.htm.

28. Neanderthal Theory, proposed by Leif Ekblad and widely distributed, http://autismnaturalvariation.blogspot.com/2006/03/review-neanderthal-theory-of-autism.html.

29. denverpost.com, "Study suggests humans mated with Neanderthals," by Karen Kaplan, Los Angeles Times, May 7, 2010. http://www.denverpost.com/nationworld/ci_15034888.

30. nytimes.com, "In a Novel Theory of Mental Disorders, Parents' Genes Are in Competition," by Benedict Carey, 11/10/2008. http://www.nytimes.com/2008/11/11/health/research/11brain.html.

31. Neuropsychologia, Grezes, J., et al. "A failure to grasp the affective meaning of actions in autism spectrum disorder subjects," 2009. doi:10.1016/j.neuropsychologia.2009.02.021 http://www.juliegrezes.com/GrezesWickerBerthozDeGelder_Neuropsychologia2009.pdf.

CRIME

1. O.A.S.I.S., "Asperger Syndrome," Stephen Bauer, M.D., MPH
www.udel.edu/bkirby/asperger/as_thru_years.html
http://www.udel.edu/bkirby/asperger/as_thru_years.html
http://www.aspergersyndrome.org/.

2. TIMESONLINE, "Teenager wings it with a fake airline," by Daniel Foggo and Martin Foley, 7/19/2009. http://business.timesonline.co.uk/tol/business/industry_sectors/transport/article6719191.ece.

3. The Independent, "'Talented' Asperger's man escapes jail for exam fraud," by Amy Caulfield, March 1, 2008. www.independent.co.uk/news/uk/crime/talented-aspergers-man-escapes-jail-for-exam-fraud-789991.html.

4. DAILY NEWS, NY, "City's great train robber at it again: Serial subway imposter caught," by Jonathan Lemire, Tanangachi Mifuni, and Larry McShane, June 14, 2008. www.nydailynews.com/news/ny_crime/2008/06/14/2008-06-14_citys_great_train_robber_at_it_again_ser.html.

5. TransitBlogger.com, Newsday, "Transit Employee Impersonator Busted Again," by Transit Blogger, 6/16/2008. http://www.transitblogger.com/crime/transit-employee-impersonator-busted-again.php.

6. Gothamist: New York City News, Food, Arts & Events, "Avid Subway Enthusiast Arrested *Again*," by Dave Hogarty, 6/14/2008. http://gothamist.com/2008//06/14/avid_subway_enthusiast_arrested_aga.php.

7. The Sydney Morning Herald, "'Big cat handler' saved from the cage," by Don Mahoney and Josephine Tovey, 9/18/2008. http://www.smh.com.au/articles/2008/09/17/1221330929873.html.

8. Media News Group: Evening Sun, "No jail sentence in child porn case," by Steve Marroni, 12/24/2008. www.eveningsun.com/ci_11302382.

9. 1010WINS.com,TM & Copyright 2008 CBS Radio Inc., "Convicted N.J. Sex Offender to Get New Trial," 6/11/2008. http://www.1010wins.com/pages/2351167.php?.

10. Lancashire Telegraph, "'TERRIBLE TWINS' GIVEN ASBO," by Peter Magill, 2/14/2008. http://archive.thisislancashire.co.uk/2008/2/14/1075289.html.

11. Newsweek, "THE PHYSICIST AND THE TORCHED SUVS," by Andrew Murr from the magazine issue dated 11//1/2004. http://www.newsweek.com/id/55579.

12. Salisbury Journal, from the Swindon Advertiser, "DRUG DEALER 'ACTING LIKE A CHILD,'" 5/28/2008. http://archive.salisburyjournal.co.uk/2008/5/28/380045.html.

13. Metrowest Daily News, "Conn. teen with autism held in assault rifle shooting," by Dustin Racioppi and Don Bond, 5/15/ 2008. http://www.metrowestdailynews.com/archive/x2118739287/Conn-teen-with-autism-held-in-assault-rifle-shooting.

14. The Shetland News, "Teen fired BB gun at folk for fun," by Pete Bevington, 9/11/2008. http://www.shetland-news.co.uk/archives/2008/news_09_2008/Teen%20fired%20BB%20gun%20at%20folk%20for%20fun.htm.

15. Herald Sun, "Family takes revenge on sex attacker," by Emily Power, 2/29/2008.
http://www.heraldsun.com.au/news/victoria/family-takes-revenge-on-sex-attacker/story-e6frf7kx-1111115672842.

16. The Daily Telegram, "Autistic man to live under supervision after child enticement charge," Maria Lockwood archive, 5//20/2008.
https://secure.forumcomm.com/?publisher_ID=37&article_id=28174 (pay for archive).

17. The Age Company Ltd., "Chemistry fan jailed over drug haul," by Kate Hagan, 12/19/2007.
http://www.theage.com.au/news/national/chemistry-fan-jailed-over-drug-haul/2007/12/18/1197740272688.html.

18. Swindon Advertiser, "Bomb-making teenager could be sectioned," by Emily Walker, 9/2/2008.
www.swindonadvertiser.co.uk/news/3638375.bomb_making_teenager_could_be_sectioned/.

19. Swindon Advertiser, "Bomb-making teenager could be sectioned," 9/2/2008.
http://www.swindonadvertiser.co.uk/news/3670500.Medical_order_on_shed___bomb_maker____/.

20. Pittsburgh Tribune-Review, "Bombs net man 5 years' probation" by Jason Cato, 7/29/2008. www.pittsburghlive.com/x/pittsburghtrib/news/cityregion/s_579925.html.

21. New Zealand news on Stuff.co.nz, "Alleged cyber crime kingpin suffers autism," 12/04/2007. http://www.stuff.co.nz/national/159286 (update, 1/1/2009).

22. guardian.co.uk, "British computer hacker faces extradition to US after court appeal fails," by Duncan Campbell, 8/29/2008. www.guardian.co.uk/technology/2008/aug/29/hacking.law.

23. p2pnet news, "Gary McKinnon's mother to Obama: Please Help!," 7/28/2009.
http://www.p2pnet.net/story/25805.

24. Japan News Review, "Man jailed for 26 years for fatal attack on group of laughing students," 3/21/2008.
http://www.japannewsreview.com/society/kyushu/kyushu/20080321page_id=4222.

25. The Star, "Manslaughter conviction after stabbing," by David Walsh, 10/11/2008. http://www.thestar.co.uk/news/Manslaughter-conviction-after-stabbing.4582510.jp.

26. The Sydney Morning Herald, "Killer had autistic disorder: court," by Jane Bunce, 2/11/2008.
http://news.smh.com.au/national/killer-had-autistic-disorder-court-20080211-1rk8.html.

27. The Canberra Times, "Judge rules Porritt didn't murder mother," by Victor Violante, 4/23/2008.
http://www.canberratimes.com.au/news/local/news/general/judge-rules-porritt-didnt-murder-mother/241945.aspx.

28. South Yorkshire Times, "Stepson stabbed woman to death," 10/8/2008. http://www.southyorkshiretimes.co.uk/news/Stepson-stabbed-woman-to-death.4571371.jp.

29. The A Register, "Wife-slaying Linux guru may have 'developmental disability,'" by Chris Williams, 7/3/2008. http://www.theregister.co.uk/2008/07/03/reiser_mentally_incompetent_claim/.

30. CBS Broadcasting, Inc., "Reiser Found Guilty Of Missing Wife's Murder," 4/29/2008. http://cbs5.com/crime/hans.resiser.verdict.2.710704.html.

31. ZDnet, "Reiser found guilty of first degree murder," by Paula Rooney, 4/28/2008. http://blogs.zdnet.com/open-source/?p=2362.

32. Psychiatric Times Newsletter, "Critical Information for the Practice of Psychaitry, James L. Knoll, IV, MD, 12/11/2009. http://www.psychiatrictimes.com/display/article/10168/1491864?CID=rss&verify=0.

ASPIES SPEAK

1. Inside the Autism Experience, "Autism and Asperger's and Hearing What You are Saying: Tips for Teachers, Bosses, Parents and Spouses," by Eileen Parker, 12/9/2009. USA www.eileenparker.com/2009/12/autismhearing/www.cozycalm.com.

2. FJ Stout, a.k.a. Fiz, WrongPlanet.net, 7/21/2009. UK http://www.wrongplanet.net/postp2300611.html&highlight=#2300611.

3. bettybarton, WrongPlanet.net, 5/19/2008. UK http://www.wrongplanet.net/postt66457.html.

4. aphonos, WrongPlanet.net, 6/30/2008. http://www.wrongplanet.net/postp1550409.html&highlight=#1550409.

5. Psychology Today, "Autism and Law Enforcement: A Plea for Understanding," Asperger's Diary by Lynne Soraya, writer with Asperger's Syndrome, 5/28/2008. http://blogs.psychologytoday.com/blog/aspergers-diary/200805/autism-and-law-enforcement-plea-understanding.

6. Asperger-4-LIfe, "sights sounds and smells," by Adrian, 7/9/2008. UK http://asperger-4-life.blogspot.com/.

7. Emoal6, WrongPlanet.net, 6/18/2008. USA http://www.wrongplanet.net/postt69380.html.

8. miniMAX, WrongPlanet.net, 12/2/2008. http://www.wrongplanet.net/postt84457.html.

9. Tracker, WrongPlanet.net, 18/6/2008. USA http://www.wrongplanet.net/postp1524168.html&highlight=1524168.

10. Sedaka, WrongPlanet.net, (two posts, same day) 9/1/2008. http://www.wrongplanet.net/postt75991.html.

11. Danielismyname, WrongPlanet.net, 9/1/2008. http://wrongplanet.net/postt75991.html.

12. Susan Jaye Graham, a.k.a. sartresue, WrongPlanet.net, 9/1/2008. http://www.wrongplanet.net/postt75991.html.

13. Angela, a.k.a. Ticker, WrongPlanet.net, 9/1/2008. http://www.wrongplanet.net/postt75991.html.

14. hiccup, WrongPlanet.net, 7/22/2008. http://www.wrongplanet.net/postt72452.html.

15. donkey, WrongPlanet.net, 8/7/2008. IRE http://www.wrongplanet.net/postt73714.html.

16. sem1precious, WrongPlanet.net, 4/19/2008. http://www.wrongplanet.net/postp1360805.html&highlight=136805.

17. ngonz, WrongPlanet.net, 5/14/2009. USA http://www.wrongplanet.net/postt98871.html.

18. GodsWonder, WrongPlanet.net, 5/31/2008. USA http://www.wrongplanet.net/postt67511.html.

19. craola, WrongPlanet.net, 5/31/2008. http://www.wrongplanet.net/postp1473751.html&highlight=#1473751.

20. obnoxiously-me, WrongPlanet.net, 5/15/2009. NOR http://www.wrongplanet.net/postt98958.html.

21. Who_Am_I, WrongPlanet.net, 5/15/2009. http://www.wrongplanet.net/postt98958.html.

22. BrixBrix, WrongPlanet.net, 6/5/2008. http://www.wrongplanet.net/postp1561820.html&highlight=#1561820.

23. flamingshorts, WrongPlanet.net, 5/10/2009. AUS http://www.wrongplanet.net/postt98557.html.

24. Angnix, WrongPlanet.net, 5/10/2009. USA http://www.wrongplanet.net/postt98557.html.

25. vimse, WrongPlanet.net, 5/15/2009. NOR http://www.wrongplanet.net/postt98958.html.

26. Papakura Courier news on Stuff.co.nz, John Harold, 7/16/2008. NZ http://www.stuff.co.nz/stuff/sundaystartimes/aukland/4619361a22396.html.

27. Rebecca_L, WrongPlanet.net, 6/22/2008. USA http://www.wrongplanet.net/postp1532408.html&highlight=#1532408.

28. hiccup, WrongPlanet.net, 7/22/2008. http://www.wrongplanet.net/postt72452.html.

29. Willard, WrongPlanet.net, 7/25/2008. USA http://www.wrongplanet.net/postt72675.html.

30. Vanilla_Slice, WrongPlanet.net, 7/11/2009. HUN http://www.wrongplanet.net/postt103128.html.

31. flamingshorts, WrongPlanet.net, 5/14/2009. http://www.wrongplanet.net/postt98557.html.

32. Aysmptotes, WrongPlanet.net, 6/19/2008. http://www.wrongplanet.net/postp1524666.html&highlight=#1524666.

33. Reclusive, WrongPlanet.net, 6/22/2008. http://www.wrongplanet.net/postp1533428.html&highlights=1533428.

34. Jael, WrongPlanet.net, 7/25/2008. http://www.wrongplanet.net/postt72675.html.

35. Alyson Bradley, Aspergers Parallel Planet, NZ http://asplanet.info/index.php?option=com_content&task=view&id=79&Itemid=125.

36. WonderWoman, WrongPlanet.net, 6/2/2008. http://www.wrongplanet.net/postt72675.html.

37. Julie Langdale, irvinetimes, 9/15/2009. http://www.irvinetimes.com/news/roundup/articles/2009/09/15/391856-julie-is-taking-a-stand-tonight/.

38. Stew54, WrongPlanet.net, 3/16/2009. http://www.wrongplanet.net/postt94863.html.

39. Charles Pierce, comment, 1/06/2009. http://www.cnewmark.com/2009/01/my-nerd-thing-and-aspergers-syndrome-.html.

40. Silke, WrongPlanet.net, 5/21/2008. http://www.wrongplanet.net/postp1447071.html&highlight=1447071.

41. Linda Jones, a.k.a. earthmom, WrongPlanet.net, 5/28/2008. http://www.wrongplanet.net/postp1468682.html&highlight=1468682.

42. Sheila Schoonmaker, (2009). "What It's Like Out There" http://sheilaschoonmaker.com/2009/06/12/What-its-like-out-there/ Last accessed 12 March 2010.

43. Linda Jones, a.k.a. earthmom, WrongPlanet.net, 5/29/2008. http://www.wrongplanet.net/postp1468682.html&hightlight=#1468682.

44. 1001 PETALS, "Asperger's Syndrome," by Athena Franks, 1/29/2009. http://1001petals.blogspot.com/2009/01/aspergers-syndrome.html.

45. Acacia, WrongPlanet.net, 1/29/2009. USA http://www.wrongplanet.net/postt89597.html.

46. AC132, WrongPlanet.net, 1/24/2009. UK http://www.wrongplanet.net/postt89145.html.

47. Pragmaticus, Daily Kos: "Reflections on Austistic Pride Day by Someone With Asperger's," 6/18/2009. http://www.dailykos.com/storyonly/2009/6/18/112848/990.

48. Pat, [information withheld by request].

49. Tim Gilbert, a.k.a. glider18. WrongPlanet.net/, 4/11/2009. USA www.wrongplanet.net/postt96268.html.

50. vulcanpastor, WrongPlanet.net/, 5/21/2008. USA http://www.wrongplanet.net/postp1448170.html&highlight=#1448170.

51. Sheila Schoonmaker, (2009). "What It's Like Out There," http://sheilaschoonmaker.com/2009/0612/what-its-like-out-there/ Last accessed 12 March 2010.

52. Roger J. Balogh, MD (Dr. Balogh is a psychiatrist who was diagnosed with Asperger's Syndrome at age 52.) Autism Support Network, "Developmental Aspects of the Asperger brain," 2009. USA http://www.autismsupportnetwork.com/news/autism-developmental-aspects-asperger-brain-876341.

53. Jeffery Serio, a.k.a. Abstract Logic, WrongPlanet.net, 7/19/2009. http://www.wrongplanet.net/postt103611.html.

54. Asperger-4-Life, "How can I help you when I can't help myself?," by Adrian, 9/4/2008. UK http://asperger-4-life.blogspot.com.

55. Tracker, WrongPlanet.net, 6/18/2008. USA http://www.wrongplanet.net/postp1524200.html&highlight=#1524200.

56. Peter Hilts, Asperger's Expert, "Social Incompetence #1 Persistence &Pain," 5/13/2009. Colorado Springs, USA http://aspergersexpert.blogspot.com/2009/05/social-incompetence-1-persistence-pain.html.

57. aulrade, WrongPlanet.net, 9/8/2007. http://www.wrongplanet.net/postt43037.html.

58. aphonos, WrongPlanet.net, 6/21/2008. http://www.wrongplanet.net/postp1532086.html&highlight=#1532086.

59. Alyson Bradley, Aspergers Parallel Planet, "The Diversity of the Autism Spectrum" NZ http://asplanet.info/index.php?option=com_content&task=view&id=79&ltemid=125.

60. Colin White, a.k.a. CWhite978, WrongPlanet.net, 6/20/2009. http://www.wrongplanet.net/postt101695.html.

61. Kathy Y. Clark, a.k.a. Kat, Big Fat Kiss, "I Think Too Much," 2/28, 2009. USA http://aboutbeautyblog.blogspot.com/2009/02/i-think-too-much.html.

62. LF Morgen, Calling Earth, "Obsessive Compulsive Disorder and Asperger's Syndrome," by Laurie Morgan, 1/13/2010. UK http://calling-earth.blogspot.com/2010/01/obsessive-compulsive-disorder-and.html.

63. Asperger-4-Life, "Aye Aye, Captain," by Adrian, 9/9/2008. UK http://asperger-4-life.blogspot.com/search/label/eye%20contact.

64. Griff, WrongPlanet.net, 2/26/2008. http://www.wrongplanet.net/postp1241286.html&highlight=1241286.

65. Elizabeth Trosper, a.k.a. Spokane_Girl, psychforums.com, 12/5/2008. http://www.psychforums.com/viewtopic.php?t=32344&postdays=0&postorder=asc&start=0.

66. Brains_&_Burgers, psychforums.com, 1/26/2009. http://www.psychforums.com/viewtopic.php?t=32344&postdays=0&postorder=asc&start=0.

67. Lofty, psychforums.com, 1/26/2009. http://www.psychforums.com/asperger-syndrome/topic32344.html.

68. Diamonddavej, a.k.a. David Jordan, Autism News: and see on YouTube, "Asperger's," Documentary about Asperger's Syndrome, http://www.youtube.com/watch?v=WAfWfsop1e0.

69. Shanti Perez, Something Awkward, "I Don't Know What to Think or Say Anymore," 7/13/2009. http://shantishanti.blogspot.com/2009/07/i-dont-know-what-to think-or-say.html[link is no longer available, try:] http://shantiperez.blogspot.com.

70. BK_G, aspergerinfo.com, 7/2/2008. BC, Canada http://www.aspergerinfo.com/forums/ubbthreads.php/ubb/showflat/Number/88129/.

71. fractalcurves, Live Journal, "Insomnia," by Evguenia Ignatova, 12/16/2009. http://fractalcurves.livejournal.com/.

72. Sheila Schoonmaker, (2008). "Single versus Double-Talk" http://sheilaschoonmaker.com/2007/02/07/single-versus-double-talk/ Last accessed 12 May, 2010.

73. Katie, WrongPlanet.net, 5/6/2009. MB CAN http://www.wrongplanet.net/postt98183.html.

74. b9, WrongPlanet.net, 5/6/2009. http://www.wrongplanet.net/postt98183.html.

75. lilopleurodon, WrongPlanet.net, 5/14/2008. http://wrongplanet.net/postp1431525.html&highlight=1431525.

76. danielismyname, WrongPlanet.net, 5/15/2008. http://www.wrongplanet.net/postp1431525.html&highlight+1431525.

77. tharn, WrongPlanet.net, 5/15/2008. USA http:www.wrongplanet.net/postp1431525.html&highlight+#1431525.

78. Willard, WrongPlanet.net, 5/7/2008. http://www.wrongplanet.net/postp1413419.html&highlights+#1413419.

79. Asperger-4-Life, "How to win friends and influence people," by Adrian, 9/3/2008. UK http://asperger-4-life.blogspot.com http://asperger-4-life.blogspot.com/search?updated-min=2008-01-01T00%3A00%3A00Z&updated-max=2009-01-01T00%3A00%3A00Z&max-results=38.

80. userg, WrongPlanet.net, 7/20/2009. http://www.wrongplanet.net/postt103694.

81. April Anjard, a.k.a. liloleme, WrongPlanet.net, 7/1/2008. USA http://www.wdrongplanet.net/postp1551148.html&highlight=#1551148.

82. curiouslittleboy, WrongPlanet.net, 7/1/2008. http://www.wrongplanet.net/postp1551148.html&highlight+#1551148.

83. Emma S. J. Walker, a.k.a. N. IRE, WrongPlanet.net, 6/26/2008. USA http:www.wrongplanet.net/postp1540678.html&highlight=#1540678.

84. nettispaghetti, WrongPlanet.net, 5/30/2008. USA http://www.wrongplanet.net/postp1473571.html&highlight=#1473571.

85. Evguenia Ignatova, a.k.a. fractalcurves, A Glimpse Into My Mind, "Asperger's and Friendships," 6/21/2009. http://fractalcurves.livejournal.com/2180.html [not available, try:] http://fractalcurves.livejournal.com/?skip=20.

86. jinxed, WrongPlanet.net, 8/23/2008. UK http://www.wrongplanet.net/postt75160.html.

87. dansa727, WrongPlanet.net, 6/28/2008. http://www.wrongplanet.net/postt70311.html.

88. JakeWilson, WrongPlanet.net, 4/17/2008. http://www.wrongplanet.net/postp1356637.html&highlight=#1356637.

89. Asperger-4-Life, "This is my love for you," by Adrian, 6/26, 2009. UK http://asperger-4-life.blogspot.com/2009/06/this-is-my-love-for-you.html.

90. Joseph Sanchez, a.k.a. malithion2, WrongPlanet.net, 7/2/2008. USA http://www.wrongplanet.net/postt70689.html.

91. ToadOfSteel, WrongPlanet.net, 7/2/2008. USA http://www.wrongplanet.net/postt70689.html.

92. Keirts, WrongPlanet.net, 1/17/2009. http://www.wrongplanet.net/postt88633.html.

93. prillix, WrongPlanet.net, 9/8/2008. http://www.wrongplanet.net/postt76755.html.

94. Tohlagos, WrongPlanet.net, 9/9/2008. http://www.wrongplanet.net/postt76755.html.

95. Eric Whalen, a.k.a. Pundit23, WrongPlanet.net, 9/9/2008. http://www.wrongplanet.net/postt76755.html.

96. Aurore, WrongPlanet.net, 9/9/2008. USA http://www.wrongplanet.netpostt76755.html.

97. Shanti Perez, Something Awkward, "I Don't Know What to Think or Say Anymore," 7/13/2009. http://shantishanti.blogspot.com/2009/07/i-dont-know-what-to think-or-say.html [link no longer available, try:] http://shantiperez.blogspot.com.

98. aspieartist, WrongPlanet.net, 9/9/2008. http://www.wrongplanet.netpostt76755.html.

99. hal9000, WrongPlanet.net, 9/9/2008. http://www.wrongplanet.net/postt76755.html.

100. Shawn Grannell, a.k.a. sgrannel, WrongPlanet.net, 9/8/2008. http://www.wrongplanet.net/postt76755.html.

101. GroovyDruid, WrongPlanet.net, 6/18/2008. http://www.wrongplanet.net/article334.html.

102. Rick Hatfield, a.k.a. rixter, WrongPlanet.net, 6/18/2008. USA http://www.wrongplanet.net/article334.html.

103. GM, WrongPlanet.net, 6/21/2008. [access to this post is unavailable].

104. Pat, [information withheld by request].

105. 866, WrongPlanet.net, 4/17/2008. USA http://www.wrongplanet.net/postp1356637.html&highlights=#.

106. Pat, [information withheld by request].

107. Shanti Perez, Something Awkward, "I Don't Know What to Think or Say Anymore, 7/13/2009. http://shantishanti.blogspot.com/2009/07/i-dont-know-what-tothink-or-say.html [link no longer available try:] http://shantiperez.blogspot.com.

108. KatieRose212, WrongPlanet.net, 4/17/2008. http://www.wrongplanet.net/postp1356637.html&highlights=#.

109. Krex, a.k.a. Denise Junk, WrongPlanet.net, 4/17/2008. http://www.wrongplanet.net/postp1356637.html&highlights=#.

110. DanteRF, WrongPlanet.net, 4/17/2008. http://www.wrongplanet.net/postp1356637.html&highlights=#.

111. Jon West, a.k.a. Hodor, WrongPlanet.net, 4/17/2008. UK http://www.wrongplanet.net/postp1356637.html&highlights=#.

112. Postperson, WrongPlanet.net, 6/10/2009. http://www.wrongplanet.net/postt100977.html.

113. Danielismyname, WrongPlanet.net, 6/10/2009. http://www.wrongplanet.net/postt100977.html.

114. Olivia Dvorak, a.k.a. poopylungstuffing, WrongPlanet.net, 6/10/2009. USA http://www.wrongplanet.net/postt100977.html.

115. oomogi, WrongPlanet.net, 6/10/2009. http://www.wrongplanet.net/postt100977.html.

116. normally_impaired, WrongPlanet.net, 6/10/2009. http://www.wrongplanet.net/postt100977.html.

117. subliculous, WrongPlanet.net, 6/10/2009. http://www.wrongplanet.net/postt100977.html.

118. ApostropheX, WrongPlanet.net, 6/19/2009. http://www.wrongplanet.net/postt100977.html.

LOOKING FORWARD

1. Peter Hilts, http://aspergersexpert.blogspot.com/.

2. Stephen Bauer, M.D., M.P.H., The Genesee Hospital, Rochester, N.Y. http://www.aspergersyndrome.org/Articles/kelley.aspx.

3. DSM-5 Development, The American Psychiatric Association, 2010. http://www.dsm5.org/ProposedRevisions/Pages/proposedrevision.aspx?rid=94.

4. Deconstructing Neurelitism: "Position Statement on the Autism Society of America," 2/7/2009. http://blog.markfoster.name/2009/02/07/position-statement-on-cooperation-with-parents/.

5. The National Autistic society, "Our Services," 2010. http://www.autism.org.uk/nas/jsp/polopoly.jsp?d=131.

6. AWARES.org, from Medical News Today, "New study will calculate number of British adults with autism," 5/9/2009. http://www.awares.org/pkgs/news/news.asp?showItemID=904&board=&bbcode=&profileCode=&section+.

7. Southern Daily Echo, "Centre to focus on adults with Asperger's," 7/26/2008. http://www.dailyecho.co.uk/news/latest/display.var.2409966.0centre_to_focus_on_adults_with_aspergers.php.

8. "The Autistic Spectrum Disorder Strategic Action Plan for Wales," see Web site for download http://wales.gov.uk/topics/childrenyoungpeople/publications/autisticspectrumdisorderplan/?lang=en.

9. Asperger Adults of Greater Washington, 2010. http://www.aagw.net/related.asp.

10. guardian.co.uk, "Aspies are far from unemployable," by SE Smith, 3/16/2010. http://www.guardian.co.uk/commentisfree/2010/mar/16/aspergers-syndrome-employment-problems.

11. guardian.co.uk, "Employing adults with autism: Don't write them off," by Louise Tickle, 10/17/2009. http://www.guardian.co.uk/money/2009/oct/17/employing-adults-with-autism.

12. msnbc Health, "Autism seen as asset, not liability, in some jobs,' by Chris Tachibana 12/8/2009. http://www.msnbc.msn.com/id/34047713/ns/health-mental-health/.

13. A Directory for Asperger Syndrome, 2/24/2010. http://www.kandi.org/aspergers/Detailed/156.html.

14. Land of My Sojourn, "An Asperger's-friendly workplace," 6/9/2009. http://landofmysojourn.wordpress.com/2009/06/09/an-aspergers-friendly-workplace/.

15. Newswire Today, "Symmetry Electronics Starts Outreach Program," 9/2/2008. http://www.newswiretoday.com/news/39179.

16. Autism Blogger, 12/15/2008. http://autism-blog.com/high-tech-clues-facial-features-cues.

17. "Second Life, 2/25/2010. http://en.wikipedia.org/wiki/Second_Life or download at http://secondlife.com/support/downloads/.

18. Insight Hypnotherapy Clinic, "Cognitive Behavioral Therapy (CBT), 2010. http://insighthypnotherapy.ie/CBT.htm.

19. Northjersey.com: "Asperger's Pilot Program," 2/26/2010. http://www.northjersey.com/news/health/85450722_Asperger_s_Pilot_Program.html.

20. The New York Times, "Students on the Spectrum'" by Abigail Sullivan Moore, 11/5/2006. http://www.nytimes.com/2006/11/05/education/edlife/traits.html?pagewanted=3&_r=1&sq=Nov.%205,%202006,%20Coaching%20Asperger&st=cse's&scp=1.

21. Dr. Jeffrey Deutsch, 2009. http://www.asplint.com/.

22. the Courier News, "Forewarned to help," by Katie Anderson, 12/27, 2009. http://www.suburbanchicagonews.com/couriernews/news/1959738,Forewarned-Alert-program_EI.122709.article.

23. SFGate "Autism: an opportunity to show and tell what you're into," 1/31/2010. http://www.sfgate.com/cgi-bin/qws/ff/qr?term=Autism%3A+An+opportunity+to+show+and+tell+what+you%27re+into&period=all&Submit=S.

24. SAGEJOURNALS *Online* "Social challenges and supports from the perspective of individuals with Asperger syndrome and other autism spectrum disabilities," by Eve Muller, 2/26/2010. http://aut.sagepub.com/cgi/content/abstract/12/2/173.

25. Asperger's Information Card, Mark Winter and Bart Vogelzang, 2006. http://www.aspergerinfo.com/ascard.htm.

26. Durham Times, "Card to help police and autism sufferers," 5/30/2009. http://www.durhamtimes.co.uk/search/?search=%22Card+to+help+police+and+autism+sufferers.

27. From the title sequence for most episodes of Star Trek, the original television series. Narrated by William Shatner. http://en.wikipedia.org/wiki/Where_no_man_has_gone_before.

616.85882 DUN
Dunne, Martha Schmidtmann
"Wait, what do you mean?" : Asperger's

04/24/24